THE U.S. AIR FORCE ACADEMY FITNESS PROGRAM FOR WOMEN

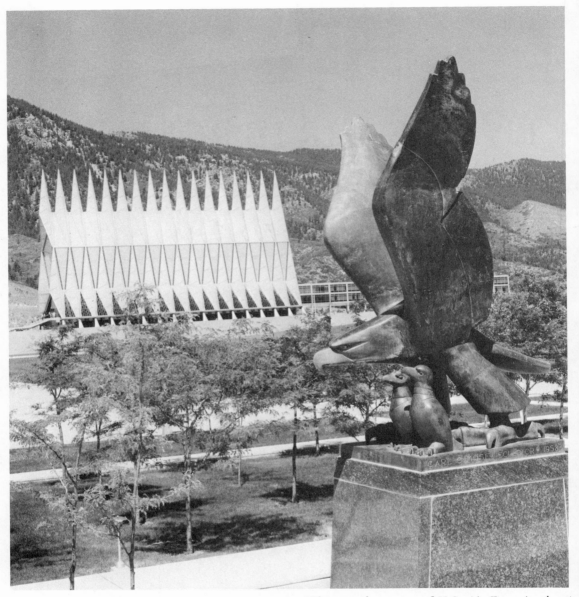

(Photograph courtesy of U.S. Air Force Academy)

THE U.S. AIR FORCE ACADEMY FITNESS PROGRAM FOR WOMEN

by Jack Galub

PRENTICE-HALL, INC., Englewood Cliffs, New Jersey

The U.S. Air Force Academy Fitness Program for Women
by Jack Galub
Copyright ©1979 by Jack Galub

10 9 8 7 6 5 4 3 2 1

Unless otherwise noted, all illustrations
are by courtesy of the U.S. Air Force Academy.

Library of Congress Cataloging in Publication Data
Galub, Jack.
The U. S. Air Force Academy fitness program for women.
Bibliography: p.
Includes index.
    1. Exercise for women. 2. Physical fitness.
I. Title.
GV482.G34   613.7'045   78-21218
ISBN 0-13-938142-2
ISBN 0-13-938134-1 pbk.

Foreword *by Colonel Don L. Peterson*

In the fall of 1976 Congress opened the doors of the military academies to women cadets. This book discusses in part the integration of the first women into the United States Air Force Academy. Some of the research material used by Jack Galub was gathered from some 18-year-old women cadets who came to the Academy in good physical condition.

We emphasize to our women cadets that physical activity is not a temporary or short-term arrangement. We want them to develop habits which will maintain them in good health throughout the remainder of their lives. We instruct them in lifetime sports such as tennis, racquetball, squash, swimming, volleyball, and badminton. Active involvement in these and other sports activities, in addition to regular conditioning programs which include running, pull-ups, push-ups, sit-ups, and standing long jump, has improved our women cadets' overall physical condition.

The minimum standards of our conditioning program are raised each year to provide an incentive to work harder at staying in top condition. In addition to attending instructional classes and taking part in conditioning programs, our women are also required to participate in a vigorous intramural program throughout the school year. You can readily see that physical conditioning is a part of everyday life at the Air Force Academy. To date our women have met the challenge.

We work with a large number of cadets and therefore take a group approach to the building of our fitness program. In interpreting the cardiovascular enhancement aspect of our work, Jack Galub has taken a more personalized approach to conditioning. Where we score our cadets by points and categories based on their performance, he shows women how to use their own body responses to exercise as a guide to building and enjoying their own programs.

A key to your success in becoming and then remaining in good condition is to develop a proper mental outlook about regular workouts. Some people offer many excuses for not staying physically fit.

Too much work, not enough time, too many meetings, all can interfere with a conditioning program. It is important to set aside a regular period of time for your workout and then keep to it: you will notice results in no time. Think positive—enjoy yourself.

A point needs to be emphasized here for women who have not exercised regularly: start your programs slowly and systematically. It is not wise to begin too quickly or to try to do too much too soon.

Being in top physical condition means that you will work better, be less fatigued, and be capable of meeting the tough demands which each new day presents. Our women cadets work hard to stay in top physical condition. Their daily routine requires it. It boils down to one thing—it is up to you to get in shape and stay in shape. You can do it if you really want to. If you have time, visit us at the Air Force Academy and see our programs in action.

Good luck in your efforts to attain "total fitness."

Don L. Peterson, Colonel, USAF
Head of the Department of Physical Education
United States Air Force Academy
Colorado Springs

Foreword *by William S. Gualtiere, Ph.D.*

The human body deteriorates with disuse or inactivity. Maintenance of the integrity of body cells, organs, and systems requires stimulation and/or movement. To appreciate the significance of this, one need only observe an individual who has been bedridden or deprived of mental stimulation for an extended period of time. Mental and physical activity, it long has been realized, go hand in hand with the healthy body. The term "healthy" here denotes quality of life rather than freedom from disease.

Industrialization has brought about a significant reduction in the activity level of most occupations and household chores. As a result, flabby muscles and overweight problems unfortunately are very much a part of the American scene.

More people today are becoming involved with physical exercise on a regular basis. Interestingly, the "exercise boom" of the Seventies is made up of women as well as men, from all age groups. It is not uncommon now to hear a woman say: "Meet you on the court in twenty minutes. Hope we have enough time to complete at least two sets." Or, "I've been jogging regularly for the past two years. More recently, I've increased my distance to where I feel ready for a marathon." Or, "Starting the day with thirty minutes of swimming is a must for me. It gives me the physical and mental set to get me through the day."

What are the reasons behind the upsurge in the number of women participating in exercise programs and sports activity? Undoubtedly, there are many. If our women clients are fairly representative of this population, the most significant cause appears to be their new active role in industry. The corporate ladder is more open to women now. Their new opportunities appear to expose them to new stresses for which many, as they soon learn, are unprepared physically and emotionally. They have found that regular, vigorous exercise helps them cope with the demands of their changing lifestyles.

Many nonworking women feel that maintaining a household requires too little energy output. They literally crave a few hours each week on the tennis court or track. In addition, many women have come to the realization—which research supports—that exercise is as beneficial as proper nutrition in maintaining an attractive figure.

Recent years have witnessed the emergence of an exercise science. Included in this body of knowledge for the beginning exerciser are principles, not all of which have been fully delineated, governing the establishment of an exercise program. In fact, today we speak in terms of writing a prescription for exercise, much in the way a physician would write a drug prescription to treat a particular disorder or disease—spelling out precisely the intensity, duration (times per session), and frequency (times per week) of exercise.

Utilization of the prescription process affords the individual maximum return on time spent exercising, while minimizing the likelihood of skeletal and neuromuscular problems and cardiovascular disorders. One must do enough, but, on the other hand, one should not overdo.

In general, the exercise prescription process involves:

1. Identifying the component of physical fitness in which improvement is desired (i.e., strength, cardiovascular [aerobic] fitness, agility, flexibility, etc.).
2. Assessing the individual's capacity relative to the specific fitness component.
3. Writing the actual prescription.
4. Carrying out the program.
5. Periodic reassessment, with subsequent adjustments in the program.

The U.S. Air Force Academy Fitness Program for Women shows the individual woman how she can apply the Air Force Academy Fitness Program to the exercise prescription process.

If you follow this program consistently, you should derive the benefits you seek.

William S. Gualtiere, Ph.D.
Director, Cardio-Metrics Institute
New York

Preface

Women have been part of the Air Force since 1948. But it wasn't until 1976 that they were accepted by the Air Force Academy as cadets.

That was a milestone. But if we step back in time to the grim days of World War II, we discover an almost forgotten group of more than 1,000 women who flew unheralded but often dangerous missions over the United States so male pilots could be freed for combat.

They were members of the Women's Airforce Service Pilots (WASP). Civilians, but wearing military uniforms and wings, they logged more than 60 million miles in Flying Fortresses and other bombers, transports and the fast, tricky fighters of that era. One woman pilot even checked out one of our first jet fighters.

The WASPs towed target sleeves behind planes to give moving targets to pilots and gunners learning to fire live ammunition. They towed gliders, ferried new planes from factories to points of embarkation and war-battered aircraft back to maintenance stations.

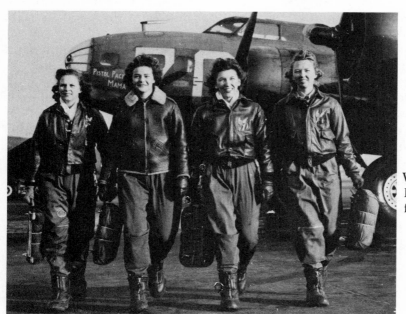

WASPs in training for B-17 Flying Fortress ferrying during World War II

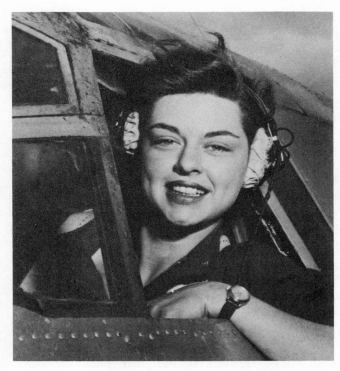

WASP ready for takeoff
on a ferry mission.

They taught male pilots to fly and to use their planes' instruments. They flight-tested just about every type of military aircraft built. They did everything expected of men but fight. When they joined the WASP, these still-civilian women expressed their willingness to go into combat. Fortunately they were never asked to fire a shot or drop a bomb in anger, but even so, their missions were hazardous and 38 were killed while helping their country to win the air war.

Ex-WASP Leonora Anderson, now a retired Air Force lieutenant colonel, reminisces that if there was a weakness in WASP training, it was in the lack of a full-scale fitness program.

"Because I had taught physical education in high school before I joined, I was put in charge of my squadron's workouts. We put in about an hour a day of jogging, stretching exercises, and marching. We really needed the same rigorous training the men went through. We all would have benefited from that."

Today the Air Force views women's need for physical fitness differently. Women cadets and officers are required to be as highly conditioned as their male counterparts. They are expected to act equally well under stress and to react just as quickly in emergencies.

The Air Force has found that physical fitness as well as professional skills are needed to lead and carry out missions successfully.

To coin a cliché, fitness is in. Every day, it seems, more women are deciding that they should exercise. They start jogging, playing tennis, or taking part in other vigorous, effort-intensive sports.

If a woman has guidance and is not overly deconditioned, her efforts may open new vistas of self-confidence and health. She can become a happier, more secure person. If she does not have proper guidance and injures herself, however, she may turn away forever from sports and exercise. That recently happened to an associate of mine. After too many years of sitting at a desk, she impulsively bought a pair of jogging shoes, did a few bends, and started jogging. She showed some restraint but little knowledge of her body's needs. Her first time out she ran one street block, walked a second, ran a third, and so on, alternating for a full half hour. That night she was in pain. The next day she was forced to see a doctor.

Her upper body musculature was found to be extremely weak. The jarring and strain of even that one brief workout was enough to bring on a number of painful problems. She was advised never to try to jog again.

That advice may have been inappropriate. She should perhaps have been told to embark upon a series of upper body toning exercises to firm her muscles. Then she and her physician would have been better able to judge whether she should take part in more vigorous activities.

The Air Force Academy total fitness program recognizes the need women have for developing and toning their entire body. The same principles, the very same exercises used by the women cadets, can be used by you to achieve similar benefits. The exercises presented here are soundly researched and tested. If done regularly—even within a limited amount of time every day—they will help you acquire the muscle tone a healthy body demands.

A major segment of the Academy's total program is devoted to cardiovascular fitness, to building stamina and endurance. Because most women are unable to devote the same amount of time as the cadets to the complete program, and because readers may be older than the cadets, a more flexible approach to cardiovascular enhancement is taken here.

By following this program, you will quickly find yourself enjoying a level of fitness you may never have considered possible.

You are shown first how to build body tone, then how to ease into programmed running, swimming, bicycling, or other activities. This approach is taken to help you minimize the possibility of muscle tears, sprains, and strains. At the start you "make haste slowly." Then, as you round into condition, you move ahead more quickly.

You will find that the book is divided into five major sections plus an appendix. The first section leads you through the Academy fitness program and the exercises the women cadets are taught. Then you are shown how to expand your program by adding cardiovascular fitness workouts.

You are shown how to write your own exercise prescriptions based upon your age-related maximum heart rate, to make certain that you obtain maximum benefit from your workouts.

But before undertaking any vigorous exercise program, you should be examined by your physician and even—especially if you are in your thirties or older—take an exercise stress test to make certain that you are not putting yourself at risk. If you have any doubt about how any aspect of the programs presented here may affect you, your physician will be able to provide the guidance you need. There should be little difficulty in modifying them to your particular needs.

If you are like most women, you will discover that the more you do, and the higher the level of fitness you attain, the more you will want to achieve. You may well find also that the "down" moods you may occasionally have become fewer and more fleeting, that your outlook on life becomes considerably more positive, that, in short you are a happier person.

Jack Galub
New York

Introduction

Women today are markedly expanding their involvement in sports, and this reflects a new and healthier self-image of their abilities as well as a shaking off of societal attitudes that had hampered them in the past.

But women are really not newcomers to sports, nor even to the martial arts. Legend tells us that Amazons had their right breasts cut off so they could use the bow more easily. Women made up a large portion of the Dahomey army before the French occupation, and were renowned for their physique and their skill in the use of weapons. In modern history, women have often played active roles in guerrilla armies and underground forces.

In America, it wasn't until after the pioneer days that women began to play a significant role in athletics. That was in the late 1800's. By the 1900's they were competing in golf, tennis, gymnastics, fencing, archery, field hockey, and other sports.

The press paid little attention to their accomplishments. Such superstars as Helen Jacobs, Alice Marble, Pauline Betz, Patty Berg, Gertrude Ederle and Mildred Didrikson Zaharias did capture the sports columns and the public's imagination for a time. Others, such as Esther Williams and Sonja Henie, went on to Hollywood.

Still, there was a tendency to underestimate the abilities of woman athletes and to doubt their femininity. In the minds of many—even including some women—there was the feeling that there is something unwomanly about being able to throw a discus or race 100 yards.

Today, happily, those attitudes have changed. Female athletes share center stage with their male counterparts. Sports pages, television, and radio report their achievements. As a result, previously non-athletic women now are running, bicycling, hiking, canoeing, hang gliding, and skiing. On the tennis courts it is not uncommon for women in their seventies to play regularly. There are older women as well as young girls on the running paths. Women and men crowd the roads with their bicycles.

Despite this upsurge in the number of women participating in athletics, only now is substantial research underway to evaluate their performance. What happens to their bodies? What special problems, if any, do they face? How will regular training affect their ability to conceive and bear children? Are there special precautions they should take to minimize the danger of injury while running, fencing, playing tennis, and taking part in other sports?

In the forefront of current research is the Air Force Academy, whose responsibility it is to turn young women into military officers. Helping women cadets to meet the extreme physical demands the Academy makes is a major objective of the Academy's Department of Physical Education. The record shows that the department's highly trained professional staff is achieving that objective with flying colors.

This book is written to show women whose bodies have lost muscle tone and become flabby how they too can benefit from the lessons learned at the Academy. Those more active women who are interested in competitive sports will find information and guidance for building their own training and conditioning programs.

Professional educators should find informative and, I trust, useful, the description of the steps taken by the Academy to build its total fitness program for women.

If you have carried over from your school and college years negative feelings about such words as "exercise," "conditioning," and "training," clear your mind of them. Remember the sheer exhilaration of those earlier days when you threw balls, ran, jumped rope, skated? This book can help you experience that wonderful feeling again, and from now on.

I am interested in your experiences and reactions. While I cannot promise to answer all letters, I assure you that yours will be read—and possibly used in another work.

J. G.

Several brand names of commercial products are mentioned in the later chapters of this book. They do not in any way imply endorsement or recommendation by the Air Force or the Air Force Academy, but are included to show the range of products and resources now available to women, and to illustrate findings by different researchers.

While portions of *The U.S. Air Force Academy Fitness Program for Women* have been read by members of the Air Force Academy and others, the responsibility for any errors or misstatements that may appear is solely mine.

J.G.

Contents

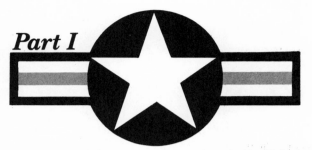

Part I

THE AIR FORCE ACADEMY TOTAL FITNESS PROGRAM

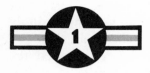

Women and the Air Force Academy

Just north of Colorado Springs, the Air Force Academy is Colorado's most popular man-built tourist attraction. Since its opening in 1958, hundreds of thousands of tourists have visited the campus, whose 18,000 acres are dominated by the spectacular peaks of the Rampart Range. Visitors are awed by the all-faith Cadet Chapel, whose seventeen sky-probing spires capture both the spirit and purpose of the Academy, and are fascinated by the planetarium and other buildings and exhibits open to the public. Of necessity, the most impressive buildings of all are off limits to the casual visitor. In them are compressed the many special facilities and classrooms needed to train cadets.

When a woman cadet graduates after four grueling years of study, she is more than a technician. In addition to the technologies of the space age, she will have studied the social sciences and humanities and will have had the opportunity to enroll in graduate-level courses that can be applied toward advanced degrees.

Still, the primary mission of the Academy is to train Air Force officers, and military instruction begins the first day the woman cadet enters. She takes part in a summer of rugged physical conditioning, survival and combat training designed to help her develop leadership qualities. Competitive sports are also an integral part of the cadets' continuing fitness program. In addition to the usual collegiate sports, women cadets learn to play squash, handball, paddleball, and golf.

Pressures on all the cadets are intense. The Academy is not a country club college at which students can take an evening off or cut class at will. There is just too much to learn and keep up with.

Since their beginnings, the nation's military academies have trained men. But like the Armed Forces themselves, they reflect changes in society, and in the past few years women have joined the previously all-male cadet ranks. Women are not expected to fight—at least not yet—but modern war is unpredictable. A woman tanker, ferry, or cargo pilot could be attacked by enemy fighters. A woman Air Police officer might find herself leading a S.W.A.T. team. And increasingly, women are being given combat-related duties in peacetime.

In the fall of 1977, for example, the Air Force opened the combat-crew missile field to female volunteers. They will carry out the same duties as men, and eventually they will be integrated into the Minuteman II program.

In early 1977 there were 40 USAF female officers commanding units ranging from small sections to a base. Less than two years later there were 60 commanders. In 1973 no USAF women were involved in aircraft maintenance; but by the end of 1977 more than 1,700 held maintenance jobs.

One outstanding champion of women in the Air Force is Antonia Handler Chayes, USAF Assistant Secretary for Manpower, Reserve Affairs and Installations. Others who have taken positions asking for more extensive use of combat-related assignments are Senator William Proxmire, Major General Jeanne Holm, USAF (Ret.), and Senator Barry Goldwater. Senator Proxmire has called for the opening of all Air Force jobs "on the basis of the individual qualifications and who can accomplish the task—not sex."

Only time will tell how far women will progress in the Air Force, but one thing is certain: as Academy graduates they will have the physical stamina and mental honing required for performing well under stress.

Don't believe all you read about push-button warfare. Combat is both physical and mental. The ride in a fighter using terrain following radar is bone shaking. Fighting on the ground—and even Air Force units could be forced to fight as infantry—calls for great mental and physical reserves. To give women cadets the physical strength, stamina, and leadership they might need in the years ahead, the Academy's total fitness program was developed.

HOW THE ACADEMY'S TOTAL FITNESS PROGRAM FOR WOMEN WAS BORN

Before the first women cadets reported for summer training in 1976, the Physical Education Department was immersed in the Women's Integration Research Project (WIRP). Its objective: To build a total fitness training program that would make it possible for the cadets to more than meet the Academy's demands of them.

The story of how the project was planned, researched, and tested is told in three reports prepared by the department task force. It reveals the care taken by the Academy to help the young women surpass their own expectations of themselves.

The total fitness program that emerged was not pieced together to make an attractive picture layout in some woman's magazine or to reflect an individual's impressions or theories. It is realistic, practical, based on thorough research and testing.

THE BIG QUESTION

One of the major questions facing the Academy dealt with women's ability to stand up to the rigorous physical demands that would be made of them during their four years as cadets. There was little thought given to showing them special consideration on the playing fields. It was felt—and, experience proved, correctly—that any easing of the demands placed on them would affect their morale as well as that of the male cadets.

Research by the Physical Education Department brought to light a considerable gap in the knowledge available about women's physical capabilities. Almost nothing was known, for example, about their ability to perform at medium altitude. That was important because the Academy sits some 7,200 feet above sea level—high enough to place extra stress on the heart and body. Also, few significant studies had been done on women's response at altitude—while at rest, during submaximal and maximal exertion, and recovery after exercise. Clearly, women were a relatively unknown quantity to serious professionals in search of factual knowledge instead of fragmentary impressions.

Considerable data were available, however, dealing with the size, form, and composition of the female body. Among the known female-male physiological differences that might make it difficult for the women to meet the Academy's male-oriented physical performance standards were:

Body Composition: On the average, women's bodies contain 8 to 10 percent more body fat than men. The male average is approximately 15 percent fat. Fatty tissue does not help body movement—it is dead weight. Women have a poorer strength-weight ratio than men, especially in the upper body. On the other hand, the fatty tissue gives women greater buoyancy in water and better protection against heat loss in cold weather, although it may prove a problem in an exceptionally hot climate.

Body Size: In general, women are about 5 to 6 inches shorter than men. Men also have some 25 pounds more body weight, giving them about five pounds more per inch of height than women. Most of this additional weight is within the bone structure and skeletal muscle. These muscles help protect the vital parts of the body, help keep blood circulation normal, and contribute to body balance, posture, and movement.

Body Structure: Women tend to have shorter legs and a broader pelvis than men. As a result, they have a lower overall center of gravity. This can be a handicap when upper body strength is required, but it does help when exercising on the horizontal balance beam.

Performance Differences: Women's ratio of heart weight to body weight is some 85 to 90 percent of men's. This implies that for a specific task, women's performance will be less than men's. They are forced to use greater amounts of energy trying to achieve comparable performance. (This is not an absolute handicap, as women who outrun men during marathons prove regularly.)

Bloodstream: A woman's bloodstream has about 15 percent less hemoglobin (a main component of the red blood cell) per milliliter of blood and 6 percent fewer red cells per cubic millimeter. As a result, women's blood has less oxygen-carrying capacity.

Capillary Network: Research indicates that women's capillary network may be less efficient than men's. So is their resistance to breakdown of capillary walls. As a result, women may bruise more easily.

Aerobic Capacity: Apparently women have some 10 to 20 percent less aerobic capacity—the ability to perform moderate sustained exercise such as jogging, hiking, or bicycling. But based on its research on women's ability to perform submaximally at medium altitude, Major Philip R. Elliott of the Academy has hypothesized that women might be less affected than men by the reduced pressure, at least during their initial exposure.

THE MORALITY FACTOR AND OTHER CULTURAL DIFFERENCES

The differences in the reactions of women to the world around them and to competitive sports offered a provocative area of research to the Women's Integration Research Project team.

There already existed a good deal of speculative writing on this subject. For example, it has been suggested the matriarchal principle emphasizes compassion and mercy while the patriarchal principle emphasizes man-made laws.

Another study of male and female values suggests women approach their duties differently from men. While women emphasize doing what seems morally right, men appear mostly concerned with achievement and advancement.

The possibility of some sex-differentiated responses to the need to win at sports also emerged from these studies. The Academy takes a competitive, will-to-win approach to both intramural and intercollegiate sports. Would women cadets have the same drive to win as men? Or would they be content with a play-well instead of a play-to-win attitude?

Research also indicated that fear of loss of feminity turned women away from sports and exercise. Cultural training and societal attitudes were blamed for these unwarranted fears.

WOMEN'S RESPONSE TO TRAINING

The study group found a paucity of research dealing with the response of women to training, especially at medium altitude. Some previously published studies suggested there would be some difficulty in their initial adjustment to altitude due to greater lung dead space and lesser breathing capacity than men. However, the reports went on, once the first hurdles are overcome, women might adjust more rapidly than men.

The Academy had learned to expect that incoming male cadets would show about a 7 percent drop in aerobic capacity due to altitude. Expectations were that women would show a similar decrease.

Studies also reported that women seem to have more difficulty in sports before the start of their menstrual cycle than during it. This was reflected in drops in performance that occurred during premenstruation. But, research also showed that higher levels of physical conditioning help women to experience less menstrual pain.

Other studies reported that women's injury rate would tend to run about double that of men for similar activities. Women showed a higher incidence of tendon, foot, and knee problems. One report pointed to short runs, sprints, and standing long jumps as the major cause of injuries among the women studied. However, it was found again that the best protection against injury is a high level of physical fitness.

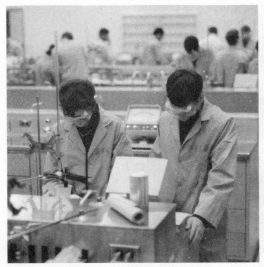

Laboratory work is an essential part of science studies at the Academy.

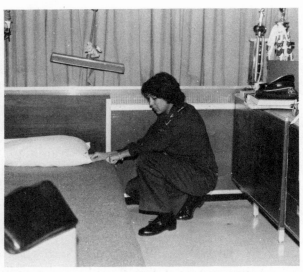

Dormitory rooms are kept neat and tidy. Cots are made up every morning before cadets leave for classroom and field work.

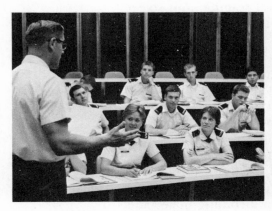

Social sciences, physics, languages and military tactics are among the classroom subjects taught at the Air Force Academy.

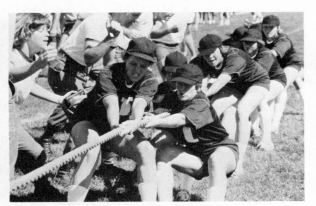

Competition between squadrons adds excitement and helps strengthen the body and the competitive spirit.

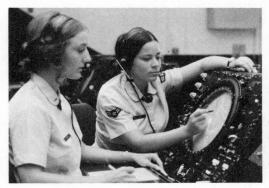

An Air Force officer and assistant direct an interceptor mission against a drone during a training exercise. This is one of the many duties for which Air Force Academy graduates are qualified after specialized schooling. Women officers may perform all Air Force duties short of actual combat.

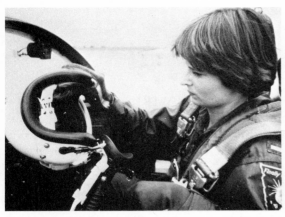

After graduation, cadets can go on to flight training if qualified.

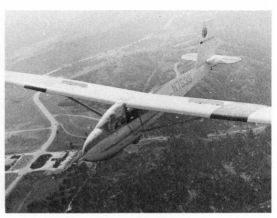

Cadets are familiarized with soaring while at the Academy.

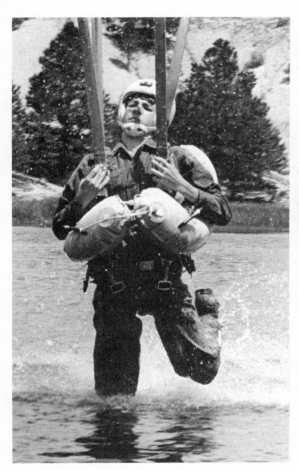

Women as well as men are taught how to ditch properly during survival training.

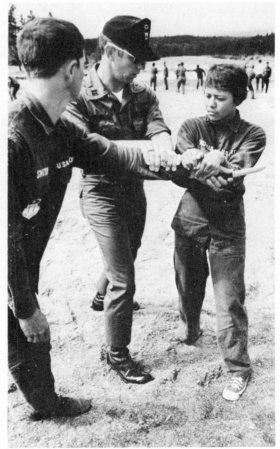

Unarmed self-defense against an aggressor is an important aspect of field training.

ATO'S TO HELP SET STANDARDS

The professional literature examined by the WIRP included studies by other military units, universities, and professional groups. But it was apparent that many of the findings might not prove applicable although they offered norms against which the cadets' performance could be measured.

As a next step, Commandant of Cadets, Brigadier General S. C. Beck, asked that a realistic physical training program be set up for fifteen young women lieutenants already in the service.

After a brief period of testing and conditioning, these women would go through a simulated Basic Cadet Summer Program and then would act as Air Training Officers (ATO's) when the first group of women cadets arrived. The ATO concept had proved successful when the Academy first opened. At that time, male officers also acting as ATO's served as surrogate upperclassmen—as example-setters—for the young cadets.

The basic cadet training given the women officers would give insights into how the young cadets might react to the intense stresses of hiking, obstacle course work, calisthenics, survival training, and athletics. Their experience would also provide valuable new information about the female body's ability to reach higher physical conditioning with training and to resist sprains, muscle pulls, and other injuries.

Before coming to the Academy, the ATO's-to-be were given a battery of four tests: flexed-arm hang for upper body strength, standing long jump to measure explosive power, volleyball throw from a kneel to measure shoulder-arm strength, and a 300-yard shuttle run for speed and anaerobic capacity—the ability to generate energy rapidly despite an inability to supply sufficient oxygen to the muscles to meet the demands being placed on them.

The last test awaiting them before they started down the same road as cadets was swimming. Each was asked to swim as far as she could in five minutes. One was afraid of water and was excused. Three covered less than 500 feet and were classified as below average. Overall the fourteen tested averaged 567 feet.

Based on national norms and other research studies, the ATO's emerged not as superjocks by any means, but as representative of the average women's population.

TAKING THE PHYSICAL FITNESS TEST

All cadets are required to take a series of physical fitness tests when entering the Academy: pull-ups, standing long jump, push-ups, sit-ups for two minutes, and 600-yard run. The ATO's took a similar test with one difference: the flexed-arm hang was substituted for pull-ups. The physical fitness levels of the fifteen ATO's proved to be in approximately the 50th percentile nationally and the mean of the first 97 women cadets applying for the class of 1980. This meant they fitted in well with the fitness levels expected for the incoming women cadets.

The last test was the equivalent of a 1½-mile aerobics run, to run as far as possible in 12 minutes. The Academy's altitude made this more difficult than usual. The ATO's averaged 1.22 miles, and after adjustments were made for altitude they were placed in Cooper's "Good Aerobic Fitness" category.

THE ATO'S START PHYSICAL CONDITIONING

Nine conditioning periods were scheduled for the ATO's for the period January 19-31, 1976. This part of their program emphasized group calisthenics, distance running, and upper body strength building. These exercises would give the Academy an idea of how well the young ATO's could meet the training goals established for the male cadets.

The calisthenics part of the program called for ten repetitions of such body tougheners as the trunk twister, side bender, push-ups, rowing exercise, three-quarter squat bender, squat stretch, and squat thrust. Like other groups of beginners from time immemorial, the ATO's didn't quite make their targets, having difficulty with the push-ups and squat thrusts. They proved slower, and had greater performance differences and more muscle soreness than entering male cadets.

One of the most effective and simplest methods of building cardiovascular fitness at altitude is group continuous running. The ATO's target was a 16-minute endurance run at an 8-minute per mile pace. Their first mile run was done in 11.5 minutes. Later they cut that time to 9.9 minutes and were able to cover 1½ miles in 14.9 minutes.

The third leg of the triad was upper body strength building. This includes regular sessions of pull-ups and wall and rope climbs.

The latter two exercises, which male cadets learn to take in stride, proved beyond the strength and skills of the women and were dropped. Later in this book, the Academy obstacle course which the women cadets have learned to run, and the civilian equivalents of the obstacle course which now are becoming popular, will be described. With training, familiarity, and conditioning, women can find them conquerable challenges.

ATO'S MOVE UP TO HIGHER PERFORMANCE LEVELS

The ATO's moved on to another phase of the physical conditioning program, this one specifically designed to meet individual fitness needs. It was understood that the same care and individual attention could not be given the cadets when they arrived, but this extra effort with the ATO's could suggest changes to be made in the cadets' program.

This phase was designed to build muscular strength and endurance as well as cardiovascular fitness. Weight training and interval running became the order of the day. Weight exercises used to improve body strength were bench press, barbell curl, leg press, military press, dead lift, straight arm pull-over, and lateral pull-down. Sit-ups supplemented the weight training sessions. Interval running sessions were used to build endurance, to bring the ATO's along to a point where they could run 3 miles in under 24 minutes.

Six weeks were devoted to this intensive work-up of the ATO's, from February 3 through March 12. At the end of the period, testing showed that the group's muscular strength overall increased 23.5 percent. There were, of course, some variables. Not all exercises showed precisely that increase, and absences had to be considered too. But in total, the results were extremely encouraging.

SPORTS ACTIVITIES—AND INJURIES

Welcome breaks in the physical education program of the ATO's were the periods devoted to track, soccer, tennis, volleyball, swimming, water polo, basketball, and gymnastics. Olympic judo competitor Major Paul Maruyama, who was in charge of the sports program, commented that the ATO's had difficulty with a number of the activities: "The ATO's were not accustomed to throwing their bodies through space for the high jump, they demonstrated a low hand-eye skill level in tennis, and their injuries appeared to be more frequent than observed with the men."

The study team's review of professional literature had prepared it for women's tendency to suffer sprains, strains, and bruises on their legs and ankles. The ATO's injuries reflected this: sprains, four; strains/pulled, four; bruises, three; and joints, one.

THE WOMEN CADETS ARRIVE

The Academy's first class of 158 women cadets—the history makers—physically made their presence felt on June 28, 1976. Those who had been raised in a military family had an idea of what to expect. For others, no matter how much they had read or heard, the reality was to prove both surprising and challenging. A military academy is unlike a civilian university. Many of the programs of study may be the same, but the objectives are different. As a result, the intensity, the demands, the expectations are greater.

Two days after their arrival—hardly enough time to learn their way around the Academy—the women started their fitness tests. Only one substitution was made in the procedures followed for men. Instead of pull-ups on an overhead bar, the women did the flexed-arm hang. On the other hand, they did regular full-body-length push-ups, not the modified exercise usually used in civilian tests.

The cadets had both motivation and youth, and their tests scores reflected their eagerness to do well before starting basic conditioning training. A comparison of their results with those of the ATO's and the norms developed by the American Association for Health, Physical Education, and Recreation (AAHPER) showed they were at a good level of fitness and ready for basic cadet training.

	Women Cadets	ATO	AAHPER
Flexed-Arm Hang	29.06 sec.	17.9 sec.	20 sec.
Long Jump	6'02"	5'10"	5'04"
Push-Ups	13.15	11.7	—
Sit-Ups	52.71	46.6	20
600-Yard Run	2:32.5 min.	2:47 min.	2:58 min.

The first cycle of conditioning got under way on July 5: breathless runs over the obstacle course (more often than not marred by falls off the overhanging ropes into the water-filled ditch), conditioning runs to build cardiovascular fitness, grass drills and physical training periods, and, for a welcome change of pace, sports. Co-ed intramural teams were organized in golf, swimming, volleyball, tennis, gymnastics, and track. The results of the conditioning runs show that the cardiovascular fitness of healthy women can be enhanced by a planned training program. Running at altitude is difficult without a preliminary period of acclimation. The air is thinner, and the heart has to work harder to keep the body fueled with oxygen. The women had an absolute minimum of acclimation, yet their running times improved and the number of dropouts on the runs decreased. The statistics for the month of July are shown in the table below:

Date	Pace	Dropouts	Distance	Pace Time	Actual Time
7/5	9 min./mile	13	1 mile	9:00	8:21
7/7	9 min./mile	4	1 mile	9:00	8:30
7/9	9 min./mile	12	1¼ mile	11:20	9:20
7/12	9 min./mile	8	1¼ mile	11:20	10:40
7/14	9 min./mile	12	1½ mile	13:30	13:15
7/16	9 min./mile	5	1½ mile	13:30	13:05
7/19	Cancelled—weather				
7/20	9 min./mile	4	2 mile	18:00	17:51

THE FIRST ACADEMIC YEAR ENDS

By the close of the first academic year in May 1977, 31 women had left the Academy, leaving 126 still in the Class of 1980. Of the 1,436 male cadets in the class, 1,099 remained. During those eleven months, the cadets took four physical fitness tests, the first immediately on arrival, and the fourth the following February. A full statistical analysis of the women's performance as well as comparisons with the male cadets' showings on the tests were made by Captain Charles P. Patton of the Physical Education Department Research Division.

Let's look at some of the mean score raw data comparing the cadets' performance on the first test with the last of the series.

- As measured by the flexed-arm hang, the women's upper body strength increased only slightly from a mean time of 29.1 seconds to a mean of 30.1 seconds. Nevertheless, their performance placed the women in the upper quartile of physically fit young women in the nation in regard to flexion strength. The male cadets did better, increasing the number of pull-ups scored from 10.8 to 11.4.

- During the first cycle, the women scored 13.2 push-ups, a measure of upper body extension strength. In February they increased the number of push-ups to 16.6, a significant 25.8 percent increase. The men raised their number of push-ups from 36.6 in the first tests to 38.5 in the final cycle.

- The standing long jump is used to measure explosive strength. The women averaged 74.8 inches initially and 75.1 inches in February. While the improvement is slight, it is meaningful. During an earlier test they had shown a drop of 3 percent in the long jump. Male cadets also improved negligibly in this test, scoring 92.9 inches initially and 93.3 inches in the last test.

- Sit-ups are an indication of abdominal strength. The women increased their number of repetitions in a two-minute period from 52.7 to 57.4. The men raised their score from 60.6 sit-ups in June to 67 in February.

- Immediately following the first four exercises, the 600-yard run was held. The women improved their mean time by 25 seconds, from 2:32.5 to 2:07.5 in February. The men's mean time also was better, dropping from 2:02.1 to 1:51.3.

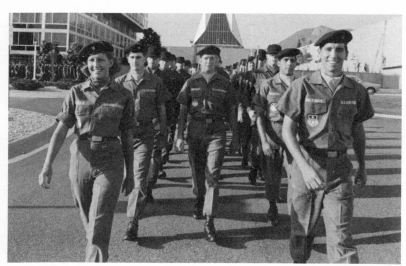

Cadets march to field training in which woman cadets take part equally with men.

A QUICK LOOK AHEAD

Today the Academy program is one of the most effective in the nation. It has proven to be practical and efficient. It does not overly depend on apparatus and can be readily followed by any woman who wishes to achieve higher levels of fitness.

Still the Academy believes women's potentials and capabilities have not been fully plumbed. It has been decided, for instance, to eliminate the flexed-arm hang as a measure of upper body strength. Instead all cadets will be asked to do the standard pull-up. The Academy is confident that women cadets, if given the chance, will show consistently better scores on the pull-up. They already are exceeding scores predicted by research.

The Department of Physical Education's confidence is reinforced by the improvement shown by the women on the obstacle course, and in particular the water jump, which is accomplished by swinging across on a rope. At first, most fell into the water-filled ditch, but as their timing improved and as their hands became accustomed to gripping the rope, they had less and less difficulty with the jump.

Just as these cadets were able to better their physical performance, so can you. You, like them, have potentials and capabilities that are yet to be plumbed. You now are on the way to doing so.

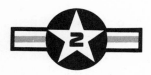

Starting Your
Total Fitness Program

Total fitness is the enhancement of the physical abilities of a woman's entire body; no longer is any segment ignored. Today, fitness is more a necessity than a matter of choice. The increased stresses women are subjected to in business, the professions, and often the home make it more vital than ever before that she be able to respond well to her environment and interpersonal relationships.

But what is total fitness? What do those words actually mean? Here are three definitions developed by members of the Department of Physical Education:

Gail Lenneville: "Physical fitness is a term used to describe the condition of the body in which the cardiovascular system, pulmonary system, and muscles operate at optimal efficiency."

Lieutenant Darlene Riding: "Physical fitness implies that level of fitness which enables individuals to carry out their daily lives in a healthful and physical manner, and have enough energy left to carry them through illness and recreation, therefore allowing everyone a different level of fitness dependent on his or her own needs and desires."

Captain Cathy Bacon: "My concept of physical fitness is a broad one—one that really implies 'total' fitness. A physically fit body is one which accomplishes its work and play harmoniously within its environment. Since mental, emotional, and spiritual fitness depend on a sound physical base, a body that is physically fit is, indeed, totally fit."

Each of these superbly conditioned women regards total fitness somewhat differently, yet what each says is similar. Their goals are the same. They view fitness holistically, as integration of the whole, the total body with the mind.

Two enthusiastic spokesmen for women's fitness, as well as for the Air Force and the opportunities it offers for careers of service and leadership, are Colonel Don L. Peterson, head of the Physical Education Department, and Colonel Thomas Moore of the Department of Athletics. Each is fully aware of the physical demands placed on women cadets and have shaped programs to meet their needs. Each also sincerely believes that physical enhancement is equally important to nonservicewomen. They believe that the fit woman is better able to achieve her full potential and success in our competitive world.

Fewer women today live Ibsen's *A Doll's House* existence. Above all else, women are saying, "We are human beings," and by the thousands they now tend their bodies with strenuous workouts that bring new sparkle to their eyes and spring to their step.

Both Thomas Moore and Don Peterson stress the importance of approaching any vigorous exercise program gradually unless you already enjoy a high level of fitness. The longer time spent arriving at a longed-for goal, the special attention given the selection of needed equipment, can help avoid the aches and strains that often are the unwelcome by-products of too much too soon.

EVERY WOMAN IS DIFFERENT

Every woman is a different chemical reactor: her body responds to training in its own way. Some condition almost overnight. They can seemingly at will run a mile or more, or play an extra set of tennis without difficulty. Others progress slowly. They must train more consistently to achieve their goals, but their successes may be all the more satisfying because of their extra effort. It is often the ex-athlete, one who has allowed herself to become deconditioned, who tries to do too much too soon. The same is true of the woman who always seems to enjoy a high level of stamina. They become careless and open themselves to injury.

EXERCISING THE AIR FORCE ACADEMY WAY

The Air Force Academy's three basic groups of exercises are designed to meet the needs of women cadets. They also can be directly used by nonservicewomen, even though they cannot devote the amount of time each day that the cadets do and they do not have the expert guidance of the Academy's professional staff.

The groups, which are described and illustrated here, are Stretching and Flexibility, Warm-Up, and Weight Training (*not* weight lifting).

Circuit Work is recommended when time available for a training session is limited. Some of the individual exercises may be familiar, some completely new. Following the Academy's exercises and doing them regularly, will tone your entire body and condition you for the more vigorous sports you will be prepared to enjoy in the days ahead.

(Demonstrating these exercises are women members of the Department of Physical Education staff.)

1. Stretching and Flexibility Exercises

(Designed by Mary Camille Maddox, Instructor, Physical Development, and demonstrated by Gail Lenneville)

These are designed to loosen, stretch, and increase the flexibility of all major muscle groups. They should be done each day you do not anticipate running, swimming, or performing another cardiovascular enhancement exercise.

If you are extremely deconditioned, start with three to five repetitions of each exercise for a period of at least two to three weeks. Try to increase the number of repetitions of each, in groups of five, until you reach 20 repetitions.

Do these exercises at a comfortable pace. Develop grace and fluidity of movement instead of speed. They are not designed to make you huff and puff. You may find one or two more difficult than others. Don't omit them; just do each more slowly.

All exercise photographs on the following pages by U.S. Air Force photographers or Jack Galub.

Circle Stretch

Stand erect, feet slightly apart. Slowly circle the head from left to back and around to forward. Then reverse direction. With one arm raised and slightly bent over the head, bend forward about 20° from the waist and slowly swing your body around in a circle from your waist up. Reverse direction with the other arm raised. Complete this exercise by slowly rotating waist and hips in an exaggerated hula-hoop motion. Reverse direction.

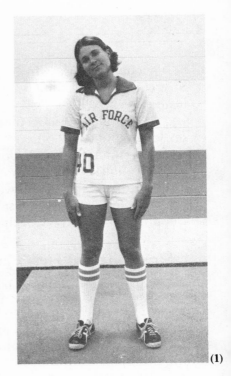

(1)

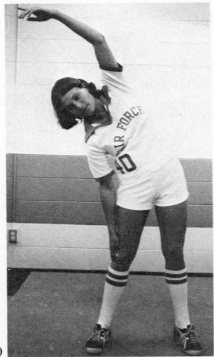

(4)

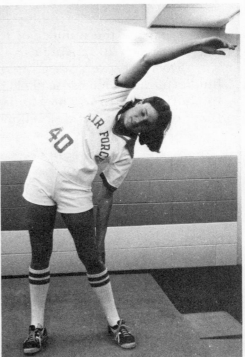

(5)

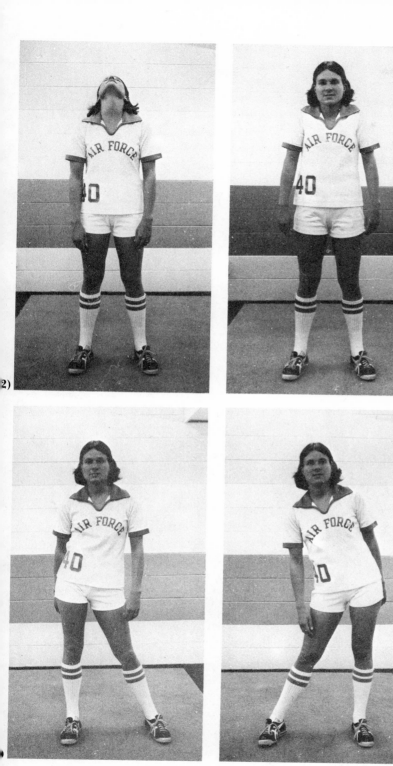

(2)

(3)

(7)

Arm Circles and Crosses

Stand erect. Raise one arm overhead. Keeping arm straight, circle overhead, then reverse direction. Repeat with other arm, then both arms together. Follow by swinging both arms so they cross in front of chest and then back behind body.

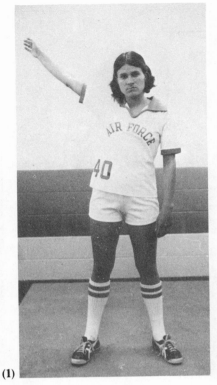

(1)

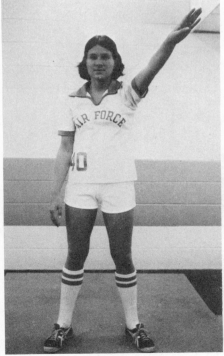

(4)

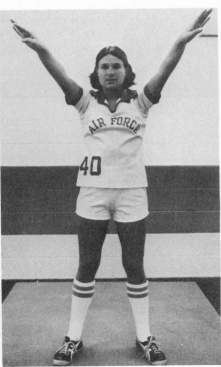

(5

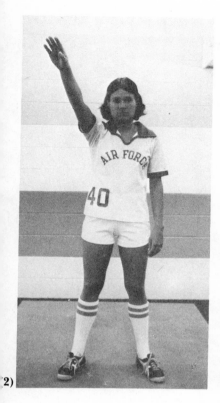

(2)

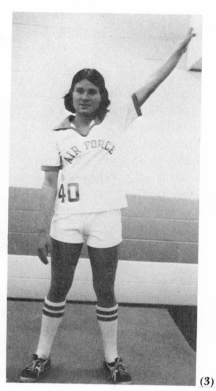

(3)

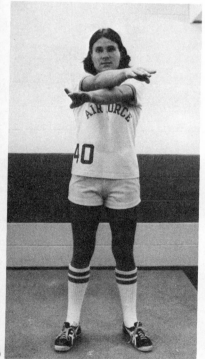

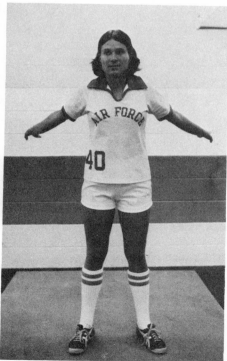

(7)

Side Bend Plié

Stand erect with your weight resting on right foot. With your right arm out-stretched at shoulder height, raise your left arm straight overhead and stretch as far as you can to your right. Then bend both knees and swing round ending with your weight resting on your left foot. Reverse arm positions and stretch to your fullest to the left.

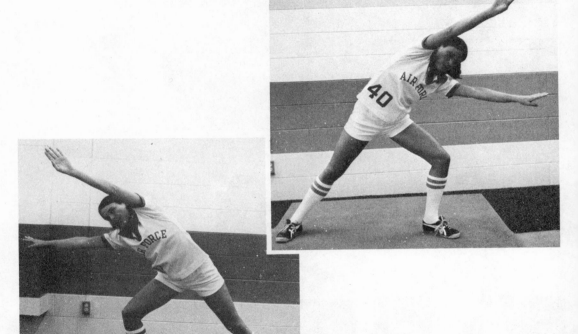

Reach, Collapse, Round Up

Stand with feet apart. Reach upward as far as you can with your right arm as you rise to the ball of the left foot. Drop arm, and repeat stretching up with your left arm while rising to the ball of the right foot. Repeat sequence three times. Then stretch up with both hands, rising to the balls of the feet. With the arms still raised, let the body bend forward bending the knees until you come to a squat. Stand up by uncoiling from the base of the spine and straightening the knees.

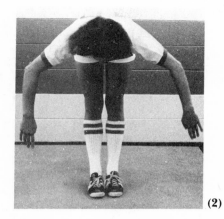

(2)

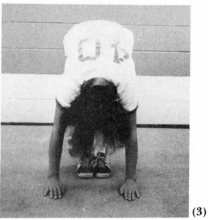

(3)

(1)

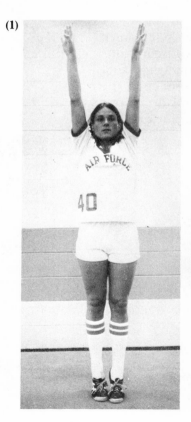

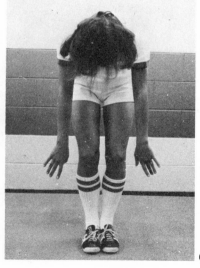

(4)

Leg Stretcher

Stand with right leg in front of left as if striding. Fully bend the right knee while arching the back with arms stretched to the rear. Then slowly lower left knee until it touches the floor while the right leg still remains forward in the lunge position. With your arms still overhead, arch the back to the rear. Straighten the body and let arms fall to the side. Bend forward as you straighten your right leg on the floor. Lean forward and touch head to right knee as you grasp your right foot. Straighten and bring your right foot back so the knee is bent as your foot rests on the floor, and your left knee remains touching the floor. Bring your left knee up and place your right foot behind with the knee touching the floor. Raise your arms and arch your body back and then come forward repeating the exercise.

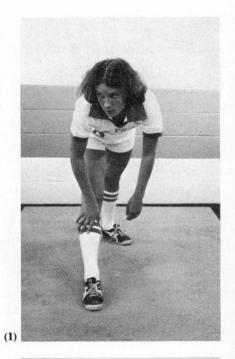

(1)

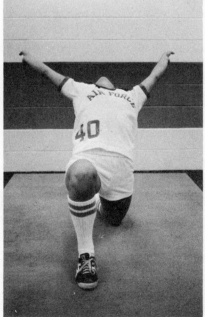

(3)

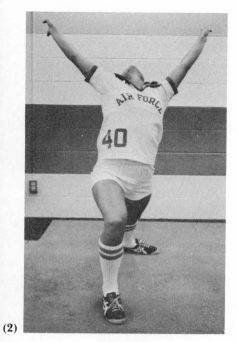

(2)

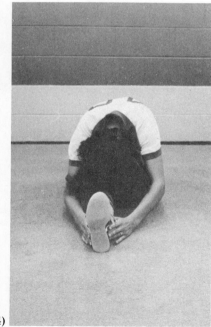

(4)

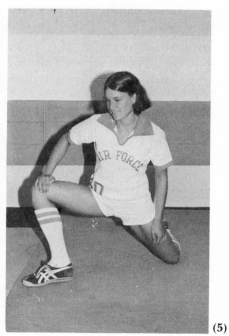

(5)

Sitting Stretches

Sit with legs stretched apart. Bend body to the right with your left hand stretched over your head to touch your right foot. Swing forward and return to your sitting position and repeat to the left side. Then sit up, bring legs together and bend forward touching head to knees. Hands should be stretched to touch feet. Roll back to the floor, bring legs back overhead and down to touch the floor behind you. Bend knees, putting shins on floor and bring knees down by ears. Straighten

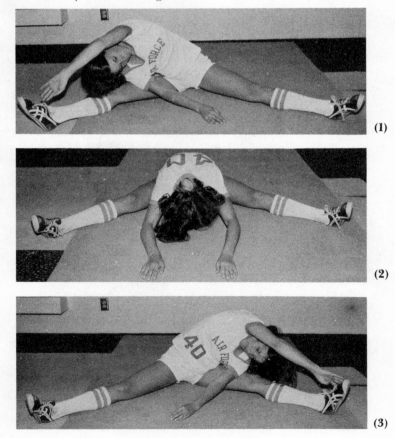

(1)

(2)

(3)

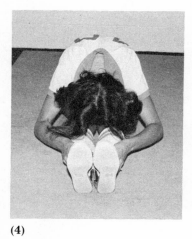

(4)

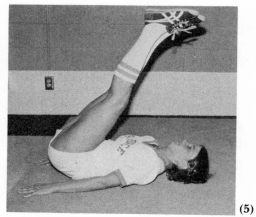

(5)

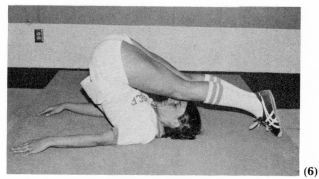

(6)

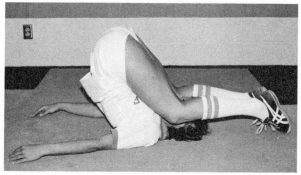

(7)

legs, swing around back up to the sitting position. Sit with both legs flexed, with the right crossed over the left. Pull the right knee to the chest by using the left arm. Twist torso to the right and press the right seat to the floor. Repeat to the opposite side. Move into the squat position. Extend right leg to the rear and press the right heel to the floor. Then repeat with the left leg. Walk both feet up to the hands, grab ankles and press head to knees while straightening legs and raising body. Then come up to a stand.

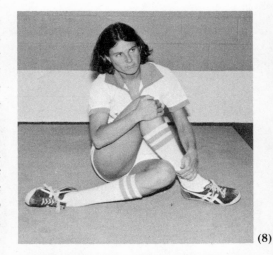

(8)

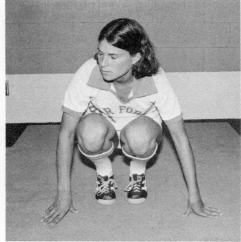

(10

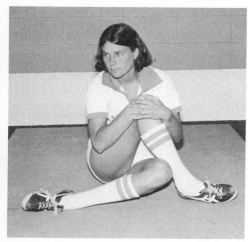

(9)

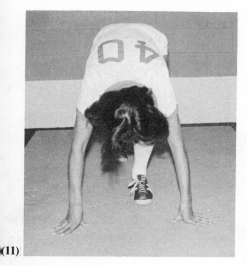

(11)

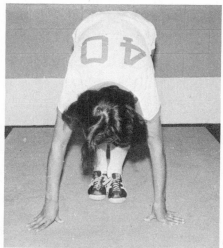

(12)

2. Warm-Up Exercises

Before starting any workout that will stress your muscles and cardiovascular system, you should take the time to warm up. These often neglected exercises "wake up" your body, increase your heartbeat rate, and pump blood through your muscles. Just as taking time to idle an engine on a cold morning will enable it to pull its load without stalling, the warm-up will help your body do its job without injury.

The warm-up exercises the Academy suggests will key up every part of the body for the running, swimming, weight lifting, or rope jumping that may await it.

Head Rotation to Stretch Neck Muscles

This exercise is the same as the Circle Stretch in the flexibility group, page 20. Do it slowly and smoothly for 15 seconds.

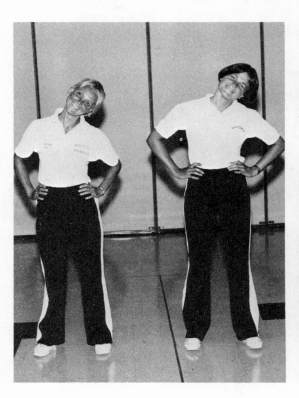 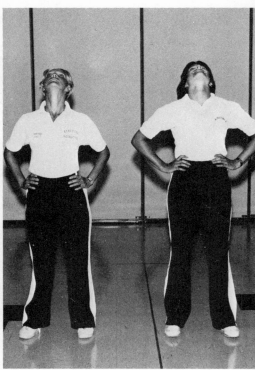

Jumping Jack

This is an all-time favorite for loosening the muscles of the arms, shoulders, and legs. Start by standing with your feet together, hands at your sides. Jump, spreading your feet apart and at the same time swinging your arms to the side and up above the head. Make certain your arms remain straight. Jump back to the starting position and repeat for 15 seconds.

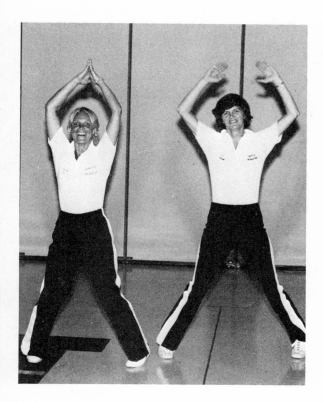

Arm Rotations

Stretch arms out to the side and rotate
them, first back, and after a number of
rotations, forward. Do for 15 seconds.

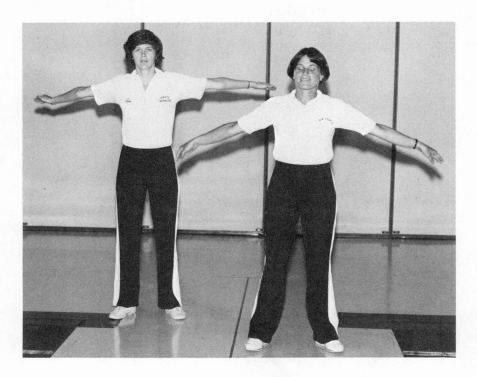

Alternate Toe Touch

Sit with legs spread apart and hands raised together overhead. Stretch slowly to the right and then left toes. Do at least 10 repetitions. This exercise stretches your hamstrings and torso as well as your shoulder muscles.

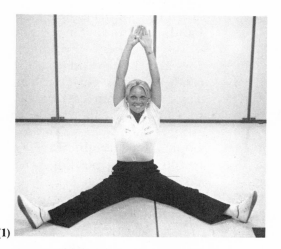

(1)

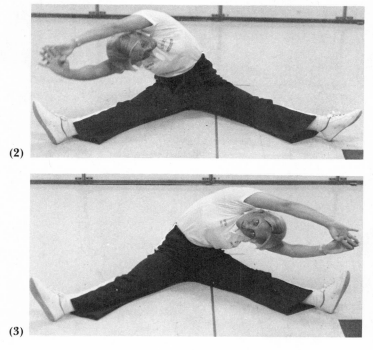

(2)

(3)

Push-Ups

You may find the normal push-up difficult to do for a week or two, but keep trying. You will succeed once your body becomes accustomed to the exercise. Extend your body on the floor keeping your arms straight. Place your hands just under and slightly outside of the shoulders with fingers pointing forward. The body should be extended so it is perfectly straight. The weight is supported by the hands and toes. Keeping the body tensed and straight, bend elbows to touch chest to floor. Then straighten arms and return to the starting position. Try not to let your stomach sag. Push-ups strengthen the arms, chest and shoulder muscles.

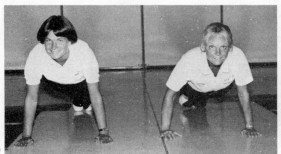
(1)

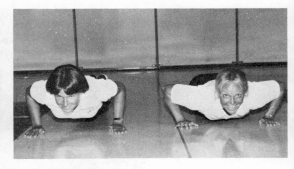

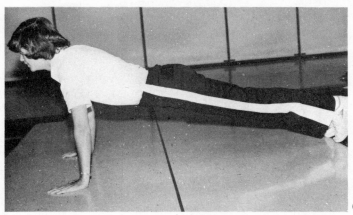
(3)

Sit-Ups (Bent Knee)

Have your legs bent at about a 90-degree angle. Either anchor your feet under a bed or chest or have a partner hold your ankles down. Each time you sit up, alternately touch your left knee with your right elbow and your right knee with your left elbow. The exercise is designed to strengthen your stomach muscles and to add flexibility to your torso. Ten repetitions.

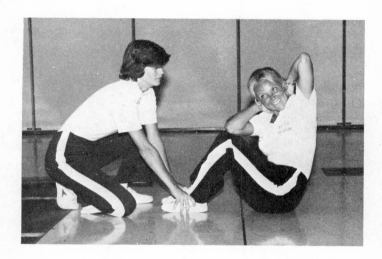

Running in Place

Even if you are running at home on a carpet, wear sneakers or jogging shoes. And, of course, make certain you lift your knees. At least two minutes at a fair pace are enough to get your heartbeat rate up.

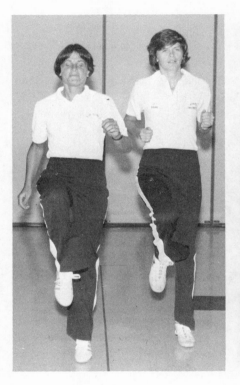
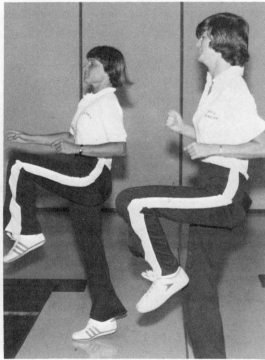

3. Weight Training Exercises
(Demonstrated by Captain Sherry Smith and First Lieutenant Darlene Riding)

The Academy recommends four basic weight exercises for upper body development. They are designed to strengthen this area, which consistently has been neglected by most exercise programs. If your physician has declared you fit for a vigorous exercise program, you should have no reluctance about starting these exercises. They cannot cause bulging muscles. Your glands won't permit that to happen.

The barbell exercises require a partner to hand you the barbell and to take it away when you are finished with the set of repetitions. Do not attempt to lift a barbell or weighted dumbbell off the floor or to set it back down while you are reclining on a bench. If you wish to lift a weight while standing, bend your knees and use your legs to give you lift power; do not bend over from the waist and pick it up. And, of course, you should wear rubber-soled shoes while working with weights to keep from slipping.

Begin with weights that are one-quarter to one-third your body weight for the bench press and bent-over rowing. For the barbell curl and military press, one-fourth of your body weight is suggested. But those suggestions are meant for young, basically well-conditioned young women in their late teens. If you are older, or even in the cadet age group, do not hesitate to start with lighter weights or to substitute weighted dumbbells for the barbell.

The secret of building strength is to start slowly and gradually and then increase weights as you progress.

Bench Press

This exercise is designed to strengthen the muscles of your chest and shoulder as well as the extensors of your arms. Lie on your back on a bench with your knees bent and feet flat on the floor. Keep feet apart so you straddle the foot of the bench.

Your partner hands you the bar, letting you hold it above your chest, arms up and elbows locked. Your hands should be placed on the bar slightly farther apart than your shoulders' width. Then lower the barbell to the middle of your chest and press or raise it back up.

The Academy suggests three groups, or three sets of six repetitions with a two-minute rest between sets. After you finish, wait three minutes before going on to the next exercise. The bench press may also be done with weighted dumbbells.

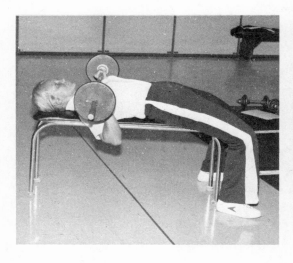
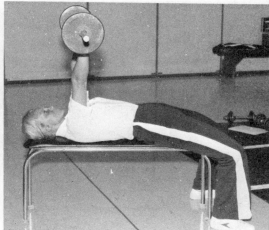

Bent-Over Rowing

This exercise will develop the muscles of your back, back of shoulders, and the front of your upper arms. Bend at the waist with the upper body at right angles to your legs. Pick up the bar or weighted dumbbells, using only your arms. Raise dumbbells to the chest and then lower them. The basic workout calls for three sets of six repetitions. Rest three minutes before going on to the next exercise.

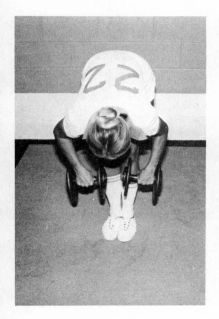 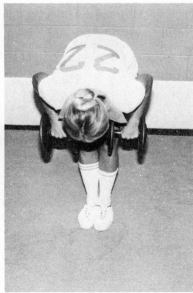

Barbell Curl

To strengthen the flexors of the arms and forearms, hold the barbell or dumbbell fully extended with a palms-out grip. Then flex your arms raising the weight to shoulder height. Keep your elbow at your side. Do three sets of six repetitions.

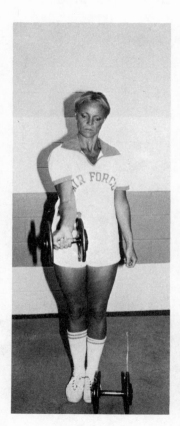 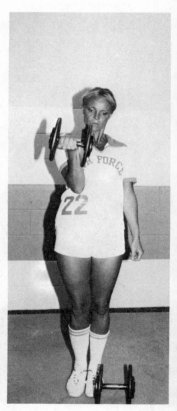

Military Press

This exercise is designed to strengthen the muscles of the shoulders, upper chest, back and the extensors of the upper arm. Stand holding the weights. First bend the elbow, pulling the dumbbell against the bicep and then straight up over the head. Do each arm alternately. Three sets of six repetitions are suggested.

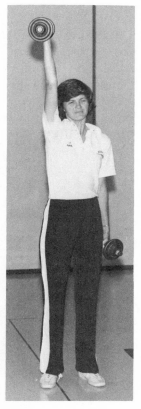

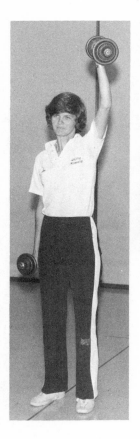

4. Circuit Workout

The circuit workout is designed to compress a maximum amount of upper body strength building and localized muscular endurance within a short period of time. These exercises are to be done rapidly.

Pull-Ups (Palms Away)

It is worth investing the $7 or so in a chinning bar so you can do pull-ups. These are the same as chin-ups, but with the palms facing forward. The Academy calls for as many as possible in 30 seconds. Make the effort and you may be able eventually to do more than you anticipate.

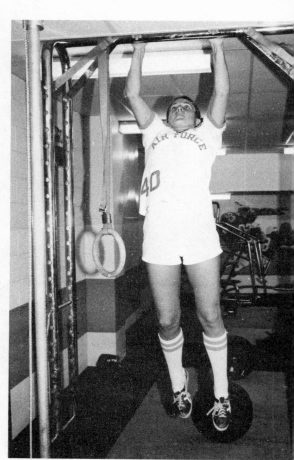

Push-Ups and Sit-Ups

These were described in the Warm-Up section. Your goal is as many as possible of each in one minute.

Dips

Dips can be done between two tables if parallel bars or a universal gym are not available. Stand between two tables that are shoulder width apart, with one hand on each table. Your elbows should be straight in the full extension position. Then bend the elbows and lower your chest to table height, and lift your body back up to the straight arm position. Your body should remain straight during the exercise. If necessary, pull your legs back at the knees so your feet do not touch the floor. Repeat as many times as possible in 30 seconds.

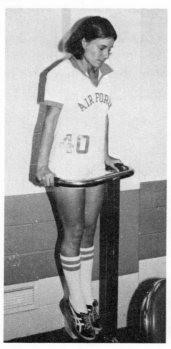
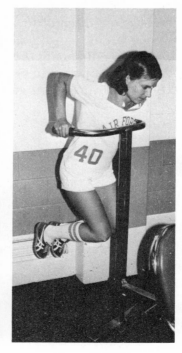

SUMMING UP QUICKLY

Let's pause and examine the meaning and importance to you of the Women's Integration Research Project and the successes of the Academy's first group of women cadets:

- With proper training and conditioning, women are able to perform well physically in many areas and activities previously closed to them.
- The reason for their previous lack of accomplishment may be traced to lack of opportunity. They seldom were permitted or encouraged, for example, to do standard push-ups, climb ropes, run obstacle courses, or take part in cross-country meets.
- Women need not fear loss of femininity through physical activity. They are protected from developing bulging muscles by their hormonal makeup. It is found that strenuous physical activity results in a firming of the body and the replacement of fatty tissue by lean tissue.
- The problem of menstruation and exercise is an old wives' tale. Women have set world records while having their period. If there is difficulty, it is probably more often during the premenstrual period when fluids accumulate. Research indicates that higher levels of conditioning tend to reduce or eliminate menstrual discomfort.
- Total fitness can be safely achieved by women who are interested in enhancing their overall level of fitness. For too many years, major muscle groups of their bodies have been ignored by their exercise programs.

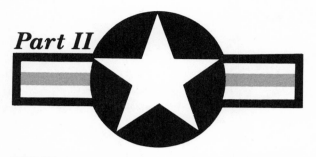

Part II

EXPANDING YOUR TOTAL FITNESS PROGRAM

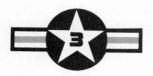

Adapting the Program to Your Needs

Done well, exercise can be fun. Every time you master a new exercise, become more proficient and skillful, you add another important marker along your road to fitness.

But there is much more to a total fitness program than stretching, warm-up, and weight training exercises. True, they help you hone your body for the stresses of everyday living and are a good morning tonic. To be truly fit, however, you should also enhance your cardiovascular and pulmonary efficiency. The Academy is well aware of this need, so a significant portion of their fitness program is comprised of running, swimming, obstacle course work, and athletics.

Your total program should include these activities as well, although your scope of activities will be more limited. There are other differences too. The Academy uses norms, fitness categories, and points to measure cadets' cardiovascular efficiency and physical performance. They take a group approach to the hundreds of young women and men they train. Cadets have professional educators, trainers, and coaches to guide and work with them. You may find yourself depending on advice picked up from other runners, swimmers, or tennis players, and their suggestions may be unsound. Cadets are issued equipment; you must select yours. They have time blocked out for athletics; you must make time.

In the next chapters, the basic precepts followed by the Air Force Academy are expanded and adapted to serve you. You are shown how you can use your age-related maximal pulse rate to set your training intensity at levels that will help you build stamina. You are given hints on buying equipment; coping with cold, heat, high altitude sickness, sunstroke, and dehydration. You are given insights into canoeing, skiing, fencing, and other activities that now are attracting increasing numbers of women.

As important as your workouts are, it is equally important that the danger of injury be minimized. Throughout, a conservative approach, a gradual building up to higher fitness levels, is stressed. Overdoing and pulled hamstrings, muscle tears, and other aches and pains go hand in hand.

Many women are now following much or all of the program outlined here. They are mentioned by name to show you that time can be made, that age need not be a handicap. Of course, age slows us down. But vigorous, consistent, enjoyable exercise more often than not takes the bite out of aging. You are able to pass the years more gracefully; you remain limber and erect while the sedentary tend to stoop and shrivel.

Common sense will suggest what you can or cannot do if you are 40 years or older. You know that the chance of outspeeding a youngster of 17 or 18 is practically nil, even though you may outlast her in a distance run if she is untrained. You know that you should also avoid unnecessary strain doing pull-ups or heavy weight lifting. There is a tendency to hold your breath at the moment of greatest strain. This causes a rise in blood pressure and increases stress. If the strain is continued during heavy lifting, the pressure in the chest increases and the amount of blood returning to the heart is decreased.

Let workouts be fun. There will be days when every ball you hit will land where you want, when you seem to float while jogging, when the laps in the pool are effortless. It is those days that will give you new insight into yourself and expand your horizons. As you heighten your fitness levels, these feelings will come more often.

You'll hate to give them up. You'll discover you are hooked on what psychiatrist Dr. William Glasser calls a positive addiction.

YOUR BEST BUY IN GOOD HEALTH

You almost always can pick out the totally fit woman from the crowd. She runs after a bus with a minimum of gasping for breath. She carries herself easily, erect. She has a smooth, quick walk. She is confident.

The fact that she is able to run three or four or more miles or swim a half dozen laps or more gives her a fuller appreciation of her capabilities, especially when she compares herself to the deconditioned men and women she knows.

Her regular exercise accelerates the flow of nutrients and oxygen-carrying blood to every part of her body. It is this oxygen that some physiologists believe helps slow the aging process. Age we must, but exercise helps us pass through the years more gracefully by keeping our cardiovascular systems at high levels of efficiency and our bodies strong and flexible. Household chores no longer may be viewed as the equivalent of vigorous exercise. Of course there is bending and lifting, but the work is not consistent enough to transform a deconditioned body into what nature intended it to be.

That is why many physicians believe that your best buy in good health is a vigorous exercise program. The effects of regular workouts are almost self-evident. After a month or two of training, you, like many others, will discover your workouts are an addiction, a way of life. If you have any doubt, listen to the chatter at the next party you go to. Young mothers who once talked mostly about schools now discuss tennis and skiing.

Once you are addicted, your major challenge is the avoidance of overproselytizing. Remember, there are still many who, like Robert Maynard Hutchins, say, "When I feel like exercising, I just lie down until the feeling goes away."

THE LONG-TERM EFFECTS OF CONDITIONING

More than 50 years of studies in human performance laboratories and research institutions have made it possible for physiologists and medical specialists to define a wide range of benefits from consistent, planned exercise. They are summarized by John R. Lasco, a physical fitness supervisor at Xerox, in a discussion of the company's executive fitness program. The program was developed to help participants achieve the following benefits:

1. Look better, feel better, and work better.
2. Improve control of weight problems.
3. Increase efficiency of heart, circulatory system, and respiratory system.
4. Lessen vulnerability to tension and stress.
5. Increase strength, endurance, and flexibility.
6. Increase ability to endure more vigorous activity with greater ease.

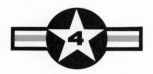

Adding CFT to Your Program

You have begun stretching, weight training, and warm-up exercises. Now you are ready for cardiovascular fitness training (CFT).

The underlying formula is simple: regular training sessions at least three times a week during which you keep your heart rate within a target zone for extended periods of time. The target is 70 to 80-85 percent of your age-related maximum heartbeat rate.*

Research has enabled physiologists to determine that 200 beats per minute (bpm) at age 20 is the maximum rate at which the heart will work. Occasionally there are reports of hearts with higher beat rates. They may be exceptions or the monitoring was not done correctly. Research also has established two additional factors you should know:

1. As you grow older, your maximum heartbeat decreases approximately one bpm with each passing year;
2. You can strengthen your heart, improve your stamina if you exercise regularly keeping your heartbeat within your target range. See Pulse Rate Table on page 54.

INTERVAL TRAINING COMES FIRST

At first you will follow an interval training formula. This calls for slow, easy effort followed by fast (stimulus) effort to raise your bpm to your target zone, then slow, easy effort again. You continue to alternate in this way (slow/fast/slow/fast/slow, etc.) until you finish your workout. As you gain strength and stamina, you will be able to gradually phase into "continuous training"; for instance, running a mile or more without having to slow to a walk periodically. Every exercise period, however, whether interval or continuous, should be preceded by a warm-up and followed by a cool-down.

*Also listen to your body. If the exercise feels moderately hard, the heartbeat range is probably correct. Increase or decrease your effort depending on how you feel.

PULSE RATE TABLE

AGE, MAXIMAL PULSE RATE (MPR), AND 70%-80% TRAINING EFFECT RANGE*

Age	MPR	70%	80%	Age	MPR	70%	80%	Age	MPR	70%	80%
20	200	140	160	39	183	128	146	58	169	118	135
21	199	139	159	40	182	127	145	59	168	117	134
22	198	138	158	41	181	126	144	60	168	117	134
23	197	137	157	41	181	126	144	61	167	116	133
24	196	137	156	43	180	126	144	62	167	116	133
25	195	136	156	44	180	126	144	63	166	116	132
26	194	135	155	45	179	125	143	64	165	115	132
27	193	135	154	46	177	123	141	65	164	114	131
28	192	134	153	47	177	123	141	66	163	114	130
29	191	133	152	48	177	123	141	67	162	113	129
30	190	133	152	49	176	123	141	68	161	112	128
31	190	133	152	50	175	122	140	69	161	112	128
32	189	132	151	51	174	121	139	70	160	112	128
33	188	131	150	52	173	121	138	71	160	112	128
34	187	130	149	53	172	120	137	72	160	112	128
35	186	130	148	54	171	119	136	73	160	112	128
36	186	130	148	55	171	119	136	74	160	112	128
37	185	129	148	56	170	119	136	75	160	112	128
38	184	128	147	57	170	119	136				

*Fractions omitted.

(Note: The formula on which this table is based is: 220 beats per minute minus age in years. According to some physiologists the formula is effective at 15 years of age. The rate tends to remain constant, in the later years unless cardiovascular disease is present. The established maximum heart rate for the various age groups can be in error 10 to 15 percent higher or lower.)

If you are at a low level of fitness, relatively inactive physically and lacking in stamina, begin with your heartbeat rate at the lower end of your target zone. As you build stamina, you will be able to raise your heart rate several beats per minute, but not to the point where you feel exhausted or ready to collapse after working out. Your workouts must be sufficiently vigorous to make you feel you are expending effort, while not straining.

There will be times when you feel you are ready to toss a coin mentally: Should you extend your sessions, or should you increase their intensity? By all means lengthen your workouts if you have the time. As you continue to build stamina, you can do both, but keep the upper level of your heartbeat range at 80 to 85 percent of your age-related pulse rate.

Should you wish to become competitive, ease into overdistance and light speed work after six months to a year of conditioning. By then you will have accustomed your heart and body to the additional stresses you will be placing on them.

YOUR CFT PRESCRIPTION

Most women find it convenient to start their CFT program with walking, jogging, or stationary bike riding. Although swimming is considered a "best exercise," many who start with that activity spend too much time chatting at poolside. On the other hand, you can watch television or read while on the bike or talk if you jog with friends.

But before you pull on your running shoes or climb aboard your in-house bicycle, rediscover the enjoyment of vigorous walking.

Your first four to five weeks of CFT will be spent walking to reaccustom your body to exercise and to tone your ankle and leg muscles for the stresses of training.

Start slowly: three to five minutes at a slow walk, followed by two minutes at a brisk pace. If you are badly deconditioned, your pulse rate will rise quickly to within 70 to 80 percent of your maximum. (Your pulse should be monitored immediately at the conclusion of every other slow-fast segment during your first several walks to make certain you are training your cardiovascular system.) After several weeks, you should discover you are able to lengthen the fast segments of your sessions and to shorten and eventually eliminate the slow segments. Gradually work your speed up to a 20-minute mile, then 18, and finally a 15-minute mile if you are able. You may find you are only able to walk the distance in 18 minutes at your very best. Accustom your body to covering the distance in that time without undue strain. If you have a friend you can walk with, all the better. If you can maintain an easy conversation while walking fast, you are not overstraining. The same principle applies to jogging.

HOW TO MONITOR YOUR PULSE

Most women find that taking the wrist pulse is a convenient method for monitoring the heartbeat. The procedure is simple if you practice at home first. If you are right-handed, first locate the pulse on the thumb side at the base of your left wrist. If you use your left hand, place the left wrist, palm side up, on the palm of your right hand, and curl the fingers of your right hand around your left wrist. Then place the fingers—not the thumb—on the pulse. Count for 10 seconds and then multiply the number of pulses by six for a full minute's reading, or refer to the pulse rate conversion table.

PULSE RATE CONVERSION TABLE

Pulse 10 secs.	Heartbeats per min.	Pulse 10 secs.	Heartbeats per min.
9	54	19	114
10	60	20	120
11	66	21	126
12	72	22	132
13	78	23	138
14	84	24	144
15	90	25	150
16	96	26	156
17	102	27	162
18	108	28	168

CFT EXERCISE PRESCRIPTIONS

These CFT prescriptions are typical of those written for women who are in good health, but deconditioned. They should be reviewed with your physician during your pretraining examination.

Remember the principles that apply to every part of this program. The warm-up/stimulus/cool-down periods should be a part of every workout, even after you have started continuous (nonstop until you cover your target distance) training. Monitor your pulse to keep from over- or under-stressing. The prescriptions that follow tell you when you should take your pulse rate. The readings should be done immediately at the end of each segment before your heart slows. After you do three or four readings, you should be able to judge by the feel of your pulse beat whether it is reading higher or lower than you are accustomed to.

The bicycle prescriptions allow you to work a bit longer during the stimulus segments. There is less stress to stationary bicycling than to running. The bicycle, not your legs, supports your body's weight.

As important as your pulse rate are your body's reactions to your training sessions. If the recommended pulse rate is too difficult to maintain, ease up. If it is too easy, increase stress slightly.

Start with the kind of exercise you find most comfortable. At the end of five or six months, after you have built up a good measure of cardiovascular fitness, you may wish to alternate between swimming and running or running and tennis, for instance. Do so. You may wake up one morning and decide you hate jogging or think rope jumping ridiculous. Don't agonize, just move on to another type of exercise— even modern dance.

But before you decide to give up jogging and start going all out on the squash court, you will need a period of conditioning to accustom your body to this new activity. So keep any pell-mell feeling you may have in check. You are in good shape, but take it easy!

Following are typical CFT prescriptions for various activities and ages. To adapt these prescriptions to your age, refer to the pulse rate table and substitute the proper target range pulse rates.

TIME (Minutes)	ACTIVITY (Intensity)	HEARTBEAT RATE (Per Minute)
ACTIVITY: JOGGING		
AGE: 25		
Warm-Up Period		
0-2	Slow walk	
2-5	Fast walk*	120-132
5-7	Walk	
7-9	Slow jogging*	132-144
9-10	Walk	
Stimulus Period		
10-12	Jogging*	150-162
12-14	Walk	
14-16	Jogging	150-162
16-18	Walk	
18-20	Jogging*	150-162
20-22	Walk	
22-24	Jogging	150-162
24-26	Walk	
26-28	Jogging*	150-162
28-30	Walk	
30-32	Jogging	150-162
32-34	Walk	
34-36	Jogging	150-162
Cool-Down Period		
36-42	Jogging—decrease speed each 2 minutes	Under 108

*Monitor pulse rate immediately on completion of exercise segment.

TIME (Minutes)	ACTIVITY (Intensity)	HEARTBEAT RATE (Per Minute)

ACTIVITY: JOGGING (*continued*)

AGE: 35

Warm-Up Period

0-2	Slow walk	
2-5	Fast walk*	114-126
5-7	Walk	
7-9	Slow jogging*	126-135

Stimulus Period

10-12	Jogging*	144-156
12-14	Walk	
14-16	Jogging	144-156
16-18	Walk	
18-20	Jogging*	144-156
20-22	Walk	
22-24	Jogging	144-156
24-26	Walk	
26-28	Jogging*	144-156
28-30	Walk	
30-32	Jogging	144-156
32-34	Walk	
34-36	Jogging	144-156

Cool-Down Period

36-42	Jogging—decrease speed each 2 minutes	Under 108

AGE: 55

Warm-Up Period

0-2	Slow walk	
2-5	Fast walk*	108-120
5-7	Walk	
7-9	Slow jogging*	120-132
9-10	Walk	

Stimulus Period

10-12	Jogging*	132-144
12-14	Walk	
14-16	Jogging	132-144
16-18	Walk	
18-20	Jogging*	132-144
20-22	Walk	
22-24	Jogging	132-144
24-26	Walk	

*Monitor pulse rate immediately on completion of exercise segment.

TIME (Minutes)	ACTIVITY (Intensity)	HEARTBEAT RATE (Per Minute)

ACTIVITY: JOGGING (*continued*)

26-28	Jogging*	132-144
28-30	Walk	
30-32	Jogging	132-144
32-34	Walk	
34-36	Jogging	132-144

Cool-Down Period

36-42	Jogging—decrease speed each 2 minutes	Under 108

ACTIVITY: STATIONARY BICYCLE

AGE: 45
(Note: Maintain steady cycling rate of approximately 13-15 mph.)

Warm-Up Period

0-2	Cycling—low tension	
2-5	Cycling—increase tension*	108-120
5-7	Walk	
7-9	Cycling—increase tension*	120-132
9-10	Walk	

Stimulus Period

10-13	Cycling-increase tension*	138-150
13-15	Walk	
15-18	Cycling	138-150
18-20	Walk	
20-23	Cycling*	138-150
23-25	Walk	
25-28	Cycling	138-150
28-30	Walk	
30-33	Cycling	138-150

Cool-Down Period

33-39	Cycling—decrease tension each 2-minute period	Under 108

AGE: 55

Warm-Up Period

0-2	Cycling—low tension	
2-5	Cycling—increase tension*	102-114
5-7	Walk	
7-9	Cycling—increase tension*	114-126
9-10	Walk	

*Monitor pulse rate immediately on completion of exercise segment.

TIME (Minutes)	ACTIVITY (Intensity)	HEARTBEAT RATE (Per Minute)

ACTIVITY: STATIONARY BICYCLE (*continued*)

Stimulus Period

10-13	Cycling—increase tension*	126-138
13-15	Walk	
15-18	Cycling	126-138
18-20	Walk	
20-23	Cycling*	126-138
23-25	Walk	
25-28	Cycling	126-138
28-30	Walk	
30-33	Cycling	126-138

Cool-Down Period

33-39	Cycling—decrease tension each 2-minute period	Under 102

*Monitor pulse rate immediately on completion of exercise segment.

PHASING INTO CONTINUOUS TRAINING

After some two months of training, you will find that you must work harder to raise your pulse to your target level. This is your body's signal that you are making progress, building stamina.

Start to shorten the length of your walking periods while increasing the intensity of your stimulus period to drive your pulse rate up to the middle or upper reaches of your target zone. Soon you will find your body moves easily along without the need for the walking periods. You are now able to begin continuous training. Most beginners are eager to reach the point where they can eliminate walking periods from their runs. Their ability to go nonstop for a quarter-mile at first, then a half-mile and eventually a mile or even a mile and a half is a high point in personal satisfaction and self-esteem.

Follow the same training pattern if you swim. Work a bit harder as you find the laps come more easily and eventually eliminate your rest periods. Should you enjoy jumping rope, and if your knees and lower legs do not bother you, increase the number of skips in each stimulus period or change your skipping style: instead of up and down work, cross the arms over your body as you skip; try making two foot contacts with every skip; swing your legs back and forth, or skip your way around the room.

Now is the time you may wish to add a second activity to your workouts. A change of pace may be refreshing as well as offer a new challenge. However, do not forget the need to keep your pulse rate within your age-related target range.

TRAINING SPECIFICITY OR TRANSFERABILITY

When you take up a new sport, you may find yourself faced with the need to retrain major muscle groups to meet new demands. Jogging or swimming, for instance, are straight-line activities using repetitive motion. Muscles are not trained to cope with the side-to-side dashes, quick turns, pivots, backward runs, and arm movements of basketball. The long-distance swimmer will not necessarily do well hiking or running. The runner's legs may quickly tire during her first games of squash.

There is a term for this lack of transferability: training specificity. However, with some practice your body can become conditioned to new activity. The more sports you learn to do well, the greater your enjoyment from exercise throughout the year. You will change from downhill to cross-country skiing to tennis to jogging as you wish.

COMPETITION

Swimmers often tire of lap after lap and join a swim club. Soon they take part in club meets. Leisurely joggers find themselves stretching their legs to keep from being passed. They start using stop watches instead of counting pulse rates. Dormant competitive urges surface.

Speed work starts. Until now you have been following a steady-state aerobic training program: your cardiovascular system has been trained to meet the steady demands of running, swimming, or bicycling done without the undue speed that leads to oxygen deprivation or the huffing and puffing of oxygen debt build up.

Theoretically your cardiovascular system is able to provide sufficient oxygen to keep your body working for long periods of time without tiring if you run, swim, or bicycle at slow to moderate speeds.

But we know perpetual motion is only a dream. The body itself also plays an important role in your activity, complementing your cardiovascular system, and sooner or later your muscles become laden with metabolic by-products that tire them. Your cardiovascular system is forced to work ever harder to make your tiring muscles respond. You acquire an increasingly larger oxygen debt. You slow down. You stop.

Speed training and overdistance work are designed to condition the body to continue fast running or swimming despite the production of lactic acids and other metabolic by-products in the muscles and the craving of the body for oxygen. The technical name for this type of speed training appropriately is anaerobic—without oxygen.

Modern training methods now help champion athletes set new records despite high levels of oxygen debt and lactic acid. The half-mile run has become little more than two extremely fast quarter-miles. Milers regularly break the four-minute mark, which is the traditional "sound barrier" of running. Just a few years ago, marathoners who finished under three hours were considered world class. Today, top-ranked women do the run in about two and a half hours.

How can you achieve competition levels of performance?

The Air Force Academy has prepared a series of coaching memorandums especially for this book that highlight their training programs. They are in Chapter 5. As you read them, bear in mind they are designed for women who plan to compete. Depending on your goals and available time, you may wish to modify their programs to meet your own specific needs.

In any event, proceed slowly and carefully to avoid injuries. Do not lose sight of your primary objective: body and cardiovascular enhancement. The goal of training is to build up, not to tear down.

SUMMING UP QUICKLY

All segments of the Air Force Academy total fitness program now are yours to benefit from:
- Stretching and flexibility exercises.
- Warm-up exercises.
- Weight training.
- Circuit work.
- Cardiovascular training, your bedrock activity.

Let us put the program into an *optimum* schedule:

- Stretching and flexibility exercises—your daily eye opener, every day.
- Warm-up exercises and cardiovascular training—three days a week. The alternate days of rest are to allow your body to rest, to shake off the early workout stiffness that should be expected.
- Warm-up exercises, weight training, and circuit workout—three days a week, alternating with the cardiovascular training.

If you are able to take an exercise stress test before starting your CFT program, by all means do so. At least have your physician give you a resting ECG if it is felt advisable.

Unless you *currently* have a marked degree of cardiovascular fitness—if you take part in school or college athletics or play tennis at least three times a week, for example—do not try to compress the exercise prescriptions given here. They are designed to show you how to bring yourself along gradually, to minimize the danger of muscle or other injury.

Listen to your pulse and your body. If you have a sprain or a cold, rest an extra day or two and then gradually ease back into your workouts. At no time should you feel you must work out if you are not well. If you are tired, however, a light workout will help dispel that washed-out feeling. That is one of the happy miracles of cardiovascular training.

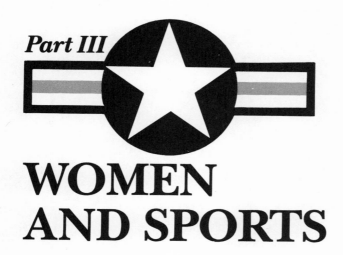

Part III

WOMEN AND SPORTS

Women and Athletics

The changing attitude of society toward women is the result to a large extent of women's own heightened understanding of what they can accomplish, not only in the home, business, and the professions, but in sports as well. The professional athlete, as well as the college and high school athlete, has helped knock down the barriers, change public attitudes, and win government support.

The 1972 Education Amendments Act includes Title IX, a key provision in the fight against sex discrimination. Under this act, the Department of Health, Education, and Welfare can deny federal funds to any institution that does not provide equal opportunity on the playing field as well as in the classroom. As a result, women now play lacrosse, soccer, softball, basketball, and track and field. At some universities there are even women rowing crews.

On their own, women runners forced such previous male bastions as the Boston Marathon to lower the barriers against them. Still holding out is the International Olympics Committee, which continues to insist that women long-distance runners cannot compete in the same run as the men.

With the clobbering of an overage Bobby Riggs by a much younger and better conditioned Billie Jean King, women's professional tennis came of age. That match may have been a promotion, but the years of steadily improving performance by women in the United States and all over the world is no myth.

In Olympic track and field, while women's winning times have been slower than men's, over the years their marks have improved steadily and impressively. In 1964 Great Britain's Ann E. Packer won the 800 meters—about a half-mile—in 2:01.1. Four years later Madeline Manning of the United States won in 2:00.9, and in 1972 Hildegard Falck of West Germany broke two minutes with 1:58.6. Then in 1976 Tatyana Kazankina of the U.S.S.R. led the field in

1:54.94. From 1928 to 1968, no women's 1,500 meters race was held. In 1972 Ludmila Bragina of the U.S.S.R. won in 4:01.4, an Olympic record and faster than marks set by six past men champions. In 1976 another Russian won the event in 4:05.45, slower but still impressive. Speedster Wilma G. Rudolph of the United States won the 100 meters in 1960 in 11.0. Armin Hary of Germany took the men's 100 that year in 10.2 seconds. Miss Rudolph was only 8/10 seconds slower than Hary. In 1976 Annegret Richter of West Germany won in 11.01. It seems inevitable that women will eventually crack the 11-second barrier. Training and motivation will prove to be the two vital factors. The talent is there.

In the United States, the people's race—the marathon—attracts women from all over the world. With the exception of a few for-women-only runs, women compete stride by stride with men over the 26-mile 385-yard distance. It wasn't always so. In 1967, Kathy Switzer, then a Syracuse University student, thought the impossible—and did it. She bundled herself in several layers of clothing to hide the curves of her body, lined up, and started the traditionally for-men-only Boston Marathon. By the fourth mile, Miss Switzer had peeled off enough of her clothing for an official to recognize that a woman had invaded that closed society and was wearing an official number. She was dragged out of the race.

That was the beginning of women's realization that they too could run the distance, learn to break through the pain barrier, and compete against men. In 1974 Miss Switzer finished first among the women running in the New York City Marathon—the Big Apple's challenge to Boston—with an impressive 3:07:29. Two years later Nancy Tighe, a 46-year-old mother of three ran the Yonkers Earth Day Marathon in 3:32 despite 50-mile-per-hour headwinds.

By 1977 the number of women trained well enough to run the marathon's full 26 miles and 385 yards had increased sharply. Ten of the 260 women in the New York City Marathon ran the distance in under three hours. Among them were Kim Merritt in 2:37:19; Miki Gorman, 2:39:11; Doris Brown-Heritage, 2:47:34; and Nina Kuscsik, 2:55:12. Of the 4,244 men in that race, according to one tally only 195 ever ran the distance faster than Miss Merritt.

Another sport that has changed dramatically in the past few years is basketball. The game as men play it is no longer man's alone. The women's genteel version has been so transformed that it is difficult for the casual onlooker to see any substantial differences between that and the men's game. No longer are women players fixed in set areas of the court. Instead they now dribble, feint, guard, pivot, lay up, and shoot with the same hard-hitting drive—in a "noncontact" sport—as men. And as with the men, tall women are starting to dominate the game. There are some marginal differences between the two games. Quarters are 10 minutes long instead of 12. The women must shoot the ball within 30 seconds of possession. The ball may be passed at will without backcourt violation. The other differences are in penalty scoring. But these differences are minor.

As a result, women are taking to the basketball court with the same eagerness that men have shown over the years. According to the National Federation for State High Schools Association, the 14,931 high schools that have women's sports report a total of 388,000 female students playing basketball. In 1971 the federation reported a total of only 294,000 women in sports programs of all kinds. As of 1978, some 1.6 million young women are taking part in high school sports.

Perhaps it is natural selection at work, but women's swimming teams have long been an integral part of American sports. After all, swimming and diving employ the same techniques whether done by men or women. Apart from the brute strength of the male swimmers, females enjoy better natural aquatic capabilities. Who can forget Gertrude Ederle's swimming of the English Channel or ignore Diana Nyad's long-distance swimming feats, or the beauty and grace Eleanor Holm and Esther Williams lent Hollywood?

Women have added lustre and excitement to professional tennis and golf. And more recently women have broken tradition and qualified as jockeys and racing car drivers.

When sports fans think of the 1972 and 1976 Olympic Games, which two competitors inevitably are talked about? None but Olga Korbut and Nadia Comaneci. Their skill and appeal successfully surmounted international and political differences in the public's mind. Miss Korbut and Miss Comaneci motivated an entire generation of American youngsters to turn to gymnastics. In 1972, when Miss Korbut won international acclaim, only about 50,000 were taking part in gymnastics. In 1978, estimates were that some 900,000 were taking part in the sport.

THE ACADEMY AND WOMEN IN ATHLETICS

Before the first woman cadet arrived at the Academy, the coaching staff was prepared for her and her needs as an athlete.

The Academy's approach to coaching women which is described below can be applied to your personal program. You probably do not have the time to practice as intensively as the cadets, but the principles they follow will help you progress rapidly and safely. The descriptions of their coaching precepts were prepared especially for your use by the Academy coaches.

It is an article of faith at the Academy that not all athletes become cadets, but all Air Force Academy cadets become athletes. Under the guidance of athletic director Colonel John Clune, the Academy's athletic program makes it possible for every cadet to enjoy athletics, whether in intercollegiate competition, intramural sports, or physical training sessions.

Eighteen intercollegiate men's and ten women's teams wear the Academy's colors. The intramural program is conducted by cadets under the supervision of the Physical Education Department. Each cadet squadron fields a team. They compete in tackle football, soccer, tennis, flickerball, boxing, wrestling, water polo, handball, squash, rugby, basketball, swimming, cross-country, team handball, volleyball, and flag football. A number of these teams are co-ed.

Underlying team games are the physical education courses taken during the cadets' four years at the Academy. The courses go far beyond the traditional 1-2-3-4 of exercise classes. They are designed to develop total body fitness, teach unarmed combat, provide instructor training, and instruct in such social sports as tennis, golf, squash, and handball.

So extensive a program demands a city of facilities, and the Academy has them. The Cadet Gymnasium boasts 24 squash courts; 19 handball courts; 6 basketball courts that have cross-court floors; 2 swimming pool areas; an indoor rifle and pistol range; gymnastics, wrestling, fencing, and boxing rooms; a supply area, and several training rooms and lockers for all cadets and coach offices. A $5.6 million field house contains a one-sixth mile indoor track (often used by the Academy faculty for running during lunch hours), an Astro-Turf infield, a basketball court with Tartan floor for varsity competition, a regulation ice hockey rink, training rooms, lockers for cadets, and administrative offices of the athletic department. In addition, there is the outdoor Falcon Stadium seating more than 46,000 spectators, 45 athletic fields spanning 143 acres for intercollegiate and intramural sports, two baseball diamonds, and a 440-meter all-weather track. Two Academy golf courses are used for varsity golf and cross-country competition.

COACHING MAKES A DIFFERENCE

While the Academy fields teams to win as does every college or university, a primary purpose of its athletic program is to train high-caliber officers. Whenever possible, female and male cadets practice and are coached together, and they often compete against one another in practice and time runs.

The success this remarkable concept of coaching has achieved is due primarily to the positive attitudes of the coaches themselves. Their approach to coaching and to working with women athletes is told by the varsity coaches in their own words:

Varsity Swimming: *Lieutenant Colonel Paul F. Arata*

The women's swimming team works from 2½ to 3½ hours each day with the workouts generally divided as follows:

Running	10-15 minutes
Weight lifting	10-15 minutes
Flexibility exercises	5-10 minutes
Swimming	2-3 hours

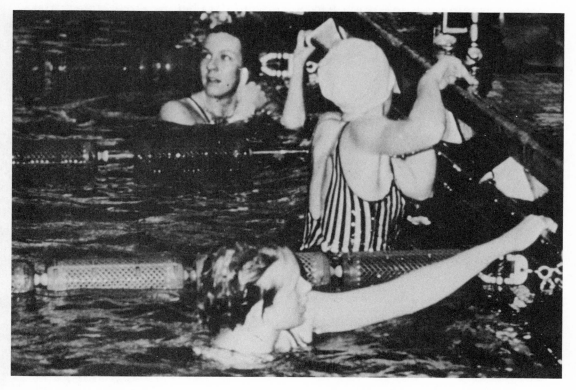

The women practice together with the men; the events and the distances covered are generally identical. They share lanes, so it is impractical to conduct separate workouts. During the first two months the swimming workouts are shorter and the dry land workouts are longer. The swimming workouts build up from 3,000 to 6,000 yards daily while the running is slowly eliminated. At the beginning of the third month, time trials take place to assess progress and the workouts are increased or changed according to the specialties of the swimmers. The distance swimmers continue to swim farther, peaking at about 11,000 yards a day. The sprinters begin quality work, including technique control along with specialization on turns.

At the beginning of the fourth month the dual season—meets with other colleges—interferes with the training program but is a welcome relief from the boredom of training. Although the basic objective is to win meets, workouts are not changed for this purpose since the long-range goals would suffer.

The intensity of the training program remains at a high level until the middle of February and throughout the entire dual meet season. A slight concession will generally be made for dual meets during January and February by reducing the distance swimmers from 11,000 yards to 6,000 yards a couple of days before a tough meet. If a chance to win the meet is extremely poor, then no concession is made and work continues as normal. This reduction is made to help spirits and to help rest the fatigued or torn-down bodies.

At the beginning of February, weight training is eliminated from the workout and flexibility exercises take place as needed on an individual basis. All efforts at this time are pointed toward qualifying for and training for the AIAW (Association for Intercollegiate Athletics for Women) Championships. Speed work becomes more and more a part of the workout, as do starts and turns. These additions to the workout are compensated for by a reduction in distance and dry land work. If illnesses aren't a factor, the first two weeks in March are devoted to being on a full smooth taper for the last big effort of the season.

The basic philosophy in training women swimmers at the Air Force Academy is identical to the philosophy for training the men.

Women's Gymnastics: *Major Carl A. Townsend*

The women's team and the men's team use the same time period and floor space for their workouts. Although the actual workout schedules are completely different, the flexibility and strength programs are similar and are often conducted together.

During the off-season (mid-August to mid-October) a greater emphasis is placed on conditioning. It takes approximately eight weeks to condition a gymnast to the level of completing a routine. The workout begins with 15 to 20 minutes of flexibility training, which is followed by two hours of workout on the equipment. During this time, the emphasis is on individual skills and short combinations. All four events are worked each day. Three days a week weight lifting is completed for 30 minutes, with a 15-minute warm-down set of exercises; during the remaining days an "on the equipment" physical conditioning circuit is used.

On-season is the second phase of workout. This period runs from mid-October to mid-April and includes the competition season. The flexibility program is continued but the weight-lifting training is stopped. The gymnasts are in good enough condition to complete a number of routines on each event each day. Prior to January, there is still some routines skill development. After January the routines are "set," with few exceptions, and now endurance needs to be developed. At this time some individuals use running, mainly sprints, some use circuits, others use large numbers of completed routines to provide

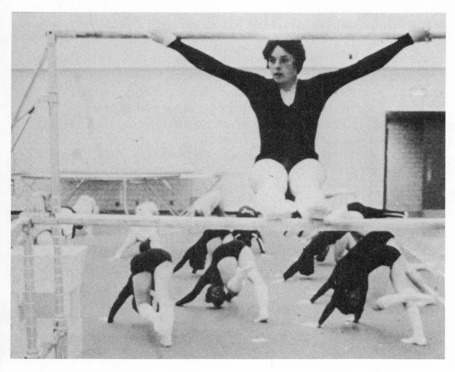

this development. Two days prior to a meet is a heavy workout day; the day before the meet is used mainly for individual skill sharpening and flexibility. The idea is to warm up the body, stretch the muscles, then warm down. This program is followed throughout the championships.

The spring training season is less organized but probably one of the most important. The coach does not have control of the gymnast's time and must work those who can make it to practice. Since the gymnast is in excellent physical condition, this time is used to learn new and more difficult skills. Little emphasis is put on total conditioning or endurance. This time is used to relearn basic skills and develop weak areas of an event. Some individuals are put on special weight-lifting programs to develop strength while others spend most of their time on flexibility or dance. During this period, there is no emphasis on training that cannot be carried over to the beginning of the next year with minimum effort during the summer.

In general, this is the same training program the men's team follows.

Women's Fencing: *Captain Todd Chirko*

The women fencers work from late August to February 28 for 2 to 2½ hours a day, Monday through Friday. The workouts vary, but at no time do the women do anything different from the men.

We begin practice with loosening up and stretches for about 20 minutes. Then we go on runs at least four times a week to strengthen leg muscles and condition for endurance. Since men's and women's legs are not used to the positions or muscles we use in fencing, we gradually go from about 30 minutes to an hour a day doing nothing but advances, retreats, and lunges with drills in between. Naturally, the runs decrease in time from an hour to half an hour as the leg work increases.

In October and November we do less running outside and more drill work with weapons inside. We are still just learning skills with the weapons. December is pretty much lost, with Christmas and finals, but we do try to have at least one competition before the break. To prepare for competition we warm up for 5 to 10 minutes, drill our legs for about 20 minutes, and fence for 1½ to 2 hours.

In January we begin again with two weeks of conditioning, mostly inside with drills on legs and fencing skills. We try to have

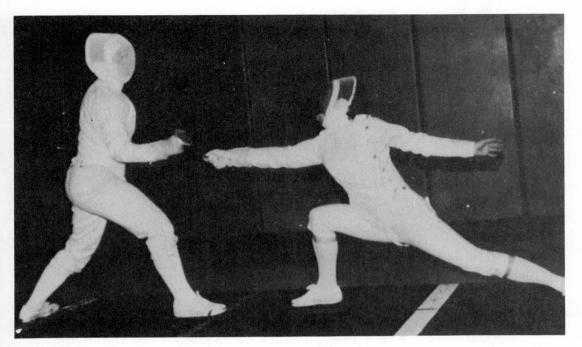

several competitions in January and February, and to prepare for these we just fence with a short initial warm-up.

Men and women are treated the same throughout the year and the women are expected to keep up with the men.

Women's Tennis: *Captain Charles Patton*

The women's tennis team is on-season in the fall (commencement of academic year until the end of October). During that period, there are a total of nine league matches in the Colorado Tennis Conference (CTC).

The workouts for the fall consist of two hours of practice Monday through Friday. On inclement weather days three indoor courts are utilized. The workouts are tailor-made to best meet the needs of the individual players. This normally consists of ground stroke, volley, service, and overhead drills. In addition, challenge matches are scheduled in order to establish a ladder and keep the players competitive.

During the spring, the team is off-season (March through the middle of May). Two-hour-a-day practice sessions are conducted, the practices closely paralleling those of the fall format. However, on inclement days, the team conducts individual conditioning workouts in the weight room and field house. All team members are required to attend all workouts.

A total of six practice matches were scheduled this past spring. These matches were utilized strictly for practice purposes, allowing all members a chance to participate under competitive conditions. However, team members' skills and tactics were corrected on the spot for added emphasis.

Women's Rifle Team: *T/Sergeant Grant Gruver*

The women on the rifle team work from 2½ to 3½ hours each day. In intercollegiate rifle competition the women compete on an equal basis with the men and the women train with the men under the same conditions.

After the team has been selected, at least two months are devoted to the instructional training phase if time permits. This instructional training includes physical conditioning, mental conditioning, rules and regulations, safety, fundamentals of marksmanship, detection and correction of errors, dry firing, and range firing.

The primary goal for the squad is to win at any level of competition. Therefore, at the conclusion of the instructional training phase, and based upon the progress of each individual as recorded in the evaluation file, teams are formulated and a concentrated effort placed on team firing. However, time must be reserved for individual firing, since a good portion of all competition is of an individual nature.

Women's Volleyball: *Captain Cathy Bacon*

The women's volleyball team workouts will generally be 1½ to 2 hours in duration. Although there will be variations, depending on the phase of our season and/or caliber of our opponents, the workouts follow this general format:

Warm-up and conditioning:	30 minutes
Drills: techniques and systems:	45-85 minutes
Warm-down:	15 minutes

During the season, the organization of our workouts will concentrate on conditioning, techniques, offensive and defensive systems, as well as strategies. The following scale depicts our areas of emphasis during the season:

Goals

1. Endurance
   Power
   Agility
2. Skill
   Form
   Mechanics
3. Viable offense and defense

4. Mental awareness

Means

Conditioning: Distance and sprint running, weights, flexibility exercises

Techniques: Serves, bumps; setting, spiking and blocking drills; dives and rolls

Systems: 4-2; 5-1; three-woman attack; crescent and W formations, middle-woman back

Strategies: Playbook (collection of plays and moves to be used in competition)

My philosophy in training and coaching the women is to encourage commitment to preparation and performance. Workouts and games are mentally and physically demanding and rewarding, thereby promoting individual growth and teamwork.

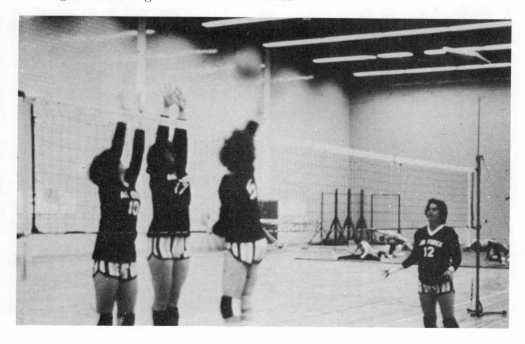

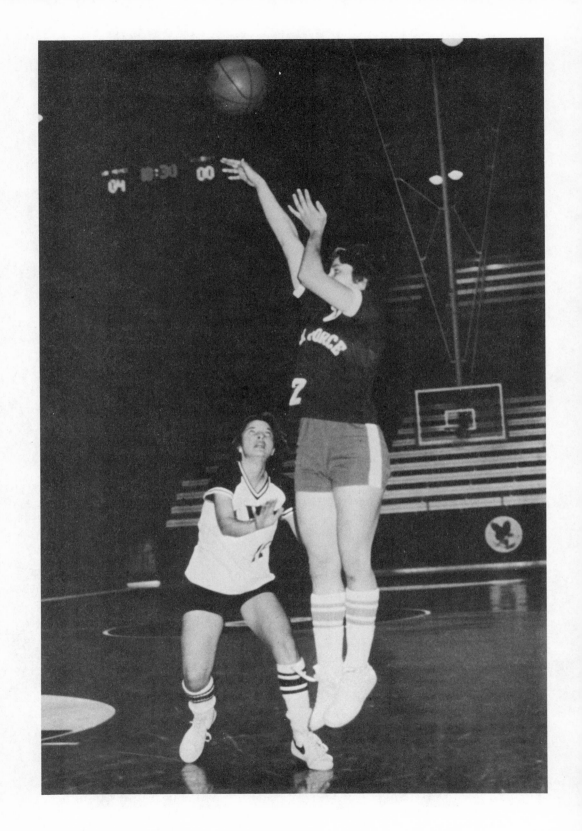

Women's Basketball: *Captain Dave Schichtle*

The women's basketball program is broken into three time periods: off-season, pre-season, and on-season.

Off-season training occurs April 1 to August 10. During this time period the women work primarily on their own. I have developed a weight program which concentrates on legs to increase jumping ability, and on arms and wrists for passing and shooting. They are encouraged to lift weights three days a week. During this time, the women run, concentrating on distance work to build endurance and leg strength. Finally, they are in the gym shooting and playing in pickup games.

The pre-season is from August 10 to December 1. This time is spent on conditioning and fundamentals. The team runs intervals from 50 to 220 yards to build endurance and speed. We then spend many hours on fundamental drills such as shooting, passing, and dribbling.

During the on-season, December 1 to April 1, the emphasis shifts from one of conditioning and skill level development to one of teamwork in which we develop our offense and defense.

Nineteen seventy-eight was the first full year this program was in operation.

Women's Track: *Captain Steve L. Miles*

The women's track team workouts are generally 1½ hours in duration. The workouts are divided as follows:

Warm-up period	10-15 minutes
Specific event workouts	60 minutes
Warm-down period	10-15 minutes

Our workouts are divided into three phases during the season. We have pre-season, early season, and competitive season conditioning. Such general conditioning is accomplished in various ways for all-around development. We do a lot of easy running, stretching exercises, and strength-building exercises. Fartlek, interval running, and weight training are the primary training methods used during this period.

In October we begin our early season conditioning program. At this time we begin to focus on perfecting form and properly executing the various techniques required for each event. We continue to develop the needed strength, endurance, and flexibility required for success in an event, but with a more intensified effort. The workouts are more intense and the athlete is exposed to longer and more strenuous training routines. The workouts may be entirely individual or may be done with a partner or in small groups. It may involve distance or speed work, or practicing jumping or throwing events.

The competitive season begins in January. During the competitive season our goal is to maintain physical condition and to sharpen the athlete's mental attitude toward competition. Our practice periods become shorter and less intense. Now we concentrate on the athlete's getting adequate rest, doing proper warm-ups, maintaining a high level of physiological fitness, and perfecting the mechanics of form.

The basic philosophy in training the women is no different from the philosophy we use for our men's program. We train together and sometimes we even compete together. The workouts for the women are very similar, in most cases the only difference being slower times for the women.

Women's Cross-Country: *Captain James E. Scott*

A typical cross-country training session consists of about ¾ to 2¼ hours of work. An approximate time breakdown is:

5-15 minutes:	Jogging ⎤
5-15 minutes:	Stretching ⎦ (warm-up)
30-90 minutes:	Running (workout)
5-15 minutes:	Jogging, walking (cool-down)

The same principles that apply to training men also apply to women, except that target times and sometimes distances need to be adjusted to women's performance levels.

At least two weeks are allotted at the beginning of the season for long-distance running with gradually increasing intensity and/or duration. Fast, explosive running is avoided at this time to allow the legs, particularly the feet and knees, to adapt to the stresses of running. This should reduce the number of injuries that occur later in the season.

Interval training is then included in the training schedule. This continues to develop cardiorespiratory endurance and, in addition, develops muscular endurance and some speed. On interval training days that involve repetitions of relatively short distances, more emphasis than usual is placed on the warm-up phase of the training session.

Various combinations of distance and interval workouts are used during most of the season, high-intensity workouts alternating with lighter ones to avoid too much psychological stress. As much variety as possible is used in location, duration, and type of workout to keep interest high and to avoid boredom. Relays and fartlek or "speed play" training are often used as variations. (Fartlek is distance running with a frequent change in pace.)

Near the end of the season, enough endurance work is continued to maintain conditioning, but more emphasis is placed on speed work to sharpen up on the timing and smoothness of running.

Women's Golf: *Major Gene Miranda*

(The program used by Coach Miranda is exactly the same for female and male members of the golf team. Every member of the team is given a folder specifically describing and illustrating a winter conditioning program for golfers. Following is an abbreviated version of that material.)

The key to this program is consistent golf-related activity throughout the winter months. There is no substitute or shortcuts to hard work. The more conscientious you are with workouts, the more efficient your swing will become. However, noticeable changes will not take place until after five or six weeks of diligent training.

The daily program is designed so it can be completed within one hour. It is very important that you budget your time so that nothing will prevent you from this one-hour workout, because deterioration of your progress will occur after a layoff of four to six days. Spring golf is too short, so do not lose what you were able to accomplish last fall.

The Winter Golf Conditioning Program

The objective of this program is not to build bulk muscle. Our main concern is to increase strength and flexibility during the period when you cannot play golf every day.

1. Start each workout by warming up with calisthenics and stretching exercises (3–4 minutes of vigorous activity is sufficient), followed by weight training.

2. *Starting Weight for Circuit:* Find your maximum weight* for each exercise, then use 60 percent of this weight as your starting point. Example: If your maximum weight for pull-downs is 100 pounds, then you will do three sets of 10 repetitions using 60 pounds.

3. *Progression:* Progress at your own pace. When the last set of an exercise becomes too easy, then increase the weight. Once you have reached 70 percent of your maximum for that exercise, then increase the number of repetitions, adding five at a time. When that becomes too easy, then increase the number of sets.

4. *The Circuit:* Start with Exercise 1 below and do one set. Then progress to Exercise 2 and do one set. Follow the sequence until you have completed all 12 exercises. Rest two minutes, then start the second set, and so on. After a few weeks you should drop the rest period between sets.

5. *The Weekly Workout*

Mon.-Wed.-Fri. *Swing weighted club 20 times.* (Start with one weight and progress to three as you get stronger).

Hit 50–100 balls.

Accomplish golf circuit on Universal Weight Machine. (Warm up with calisthenics and stretching first.)

Hang from horizontal bar. (Always finish your workouts by hanging from a horizontal bar. Try to relax your body. Hang 60 seconds, rest 60 seconds, then hang for 60 seconds again.)

Tue.-Thurs. *Swing weighted club 20 times.*

Hit 150–200 balls.

Practice putting and chip to bucket for 10 minutes.

Accomplish wrist roll exercise, 2 sets of 10 repetitions.

Run 2 miles at an 8-minute pace.

Sat.-Sun. *Play if weather permits.* (If weather is bad, hit balls, work on short game. Outside if possible.)

Run 2 miles at an 8-minute pace..

*Usually "maximum weight" is determined by trial and error. If you are not overweight and are reasonably strong for your age, your body weight corresponds approximately to your strength. As a start weights used should be no more than one-third to one-fourth of your body weight. After the correct movements are mastered, gradually add weights or plates used for training.

Exercises

(The exercises listed here were selected for use with the Universal Weight Machine. Of course, they can be done on other exercise machines if access is available.)

1. Bent-over rowing
2. Regular leg press
3. Bench press
4. Double leg curl
5. Back pull-down
6. Straight sit-up
7. Side bend
8. Golfer's exercise
9. Wrist curl
10. Forward shoulder press
11. Hip flexor
12. Double arm curl and reverse arm curl

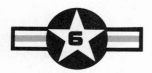

The Basic Sports

For cadets, sports is more than running around or swatting a ball. Athletics and competition add spice to their fitness program. They also inculcate lifelong fitness habits, making it simple for the young women to remain fit when they go into active duty or return to civilian life later.

You can easily develop the same helpful habits by becoming actively involved in a sport. Joining a club or a group makes that involvement more interesting and exciting.

Walking can lead to hiking and even backpacking along the Appalachian and Sierra Trails. Perhaps you never thought of skiing. Now you may ask yourself, why not? If you take up cross-country skiing, you will find your heart working harder than it did in your exercise program, but now you will have a bedrock of stamina and fitness to build on. Even a relatively simple sport, jogging for instance, can become more complex. You may decide to build up to marathon running, join a Road Runner or other athletic club. Simple lake canoeing can be upgraded into kayaking or canoe camping.

Every sport entails some degree of specific conditioning. This section covers some of the major activities you may wish to consider and the techniques involved. But to start at the beginning, you must consider posture.

GOOD POSTURE

Good posture is fundamental to everything we do: breathing, sitting, standing, walking, running, skiing. Poor posture hampers our breathing, reduces lung capacity, creates muscle imbalances, may cause bad backs and a variety of other physical problems.

Good posture calls for the easy, not stiff, carrying of the body—feet, legs, hips, trunk, shoulders, and head—in a straight line. From

85

the side when standing, the line should run through the earlobe, tip of the shoulder, middle of the hip, just back of the kneecap, and just in front of the anklebone. Hips are a reliable indicator of good posture. They should rest squarely upon the legs without tilting forward or backward.

Flabby abdominal muscles and excess weight lead to poor posture. Muscle weakness allows internal organs to sag. The abdomen protrudes, the pelvis tilts forward, the curve of the lower back is accentuated. The overweight woman's abdomen upsets her center of gravity, so she compensates by leaning back and bending her knees.

Dr. Catherine Kenney Carlton, a Fort Worth osteopathic physician, lists a number of habits that contribute to poor posture among women. Among then are holding the telephone between the shoulder and ear; sleeping prone; holding the head to one side to see around long hair, tossing long hair from side to side, much as a horse tosses his mane; wearing a too-tight brassiere, empire waistline, or high, tight belts; watching television or reading in bed with the head propped up; and sitting or lying propped up on one elbow.

Dr. Jeanne R. Pamilla, assistant attending orthopedic surgeon at the Hospital for Special Surgery at Cornell Medical Center in New York, recommends a number of exercises to improve posture. These will gradually strengthen the abdominal muscles and stretch the Achilles tendons, leg muscles, and hamstrings. She urges that they be done slowly, starting with 5 repetitions each day and gradually building up to 20 a day:

1. Stand with your back against the side of a doorway. Place heels about 4 inches from the frame. Take a deep breath, relax. Press the small of your back against the frame. Tighten stomach and buttocks, allowing your knees to bend slightly, then press your neck up against the doorway. Raise your arms to shoulder height and press both hands against the opposite side of the doorway so that your lower spine is pressed back against the door frame. Straighten both knees. Hold for 2 seconds; relax.

2. Lie on your back with knees bent and hands clasped behind your neck. Keep feet flat on the floor. Take a deep breath and relax. Press the small of the back against the floor and tighten stomach and buttock muscles so that your lower back flattens against the floor. Hold for 5 seconds; relax.

3. Lie on your back with your knees bent, feet on the floor, and your hands at your sides. Grasp one knee with both hands and pull as

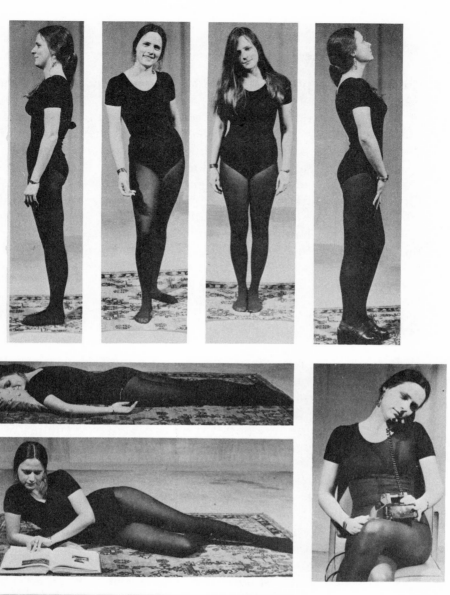
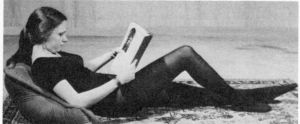

Eight common faults of posture. Clock-wise, from top left: a too-tight bra; Venus de Milo stance; craning neck to see around long hair; platform shoes; shouldering telephone receiver; craning neck to read while on back; supporting upper body on one arm; sleeping on stomach. Demonstrated by Jane Carlton. (*Source: Catherine Carlton, D.O.*)

close to chest as possible. Return leg to starting position. Repeat with other leg. Alternate.

4. Lie on your back as in Exercise 3. Grasp both knees and pull them as close to your chest as possible. Hold for 3 seconds, then return them to starting position. Straighten legs, relax, and repeat.

5. For the Achilles: Stand 2 feet from a wall, facing the wall, and place both hands at shoulder height against it. Flex the elbows and lean forward; then push back as though you are doing standing push-ups. The heels should be planted solidly on the floor during the exercise.

6. For the hamstrings: Stand erect and place one leg on a table that is about hip-high. Lean forward, stretching with both arms toward your toes. After several repetitions, place your other leg on the table and repeat.

WALKING

Walking is an easy, effective exercise offering unlimited stores of pleasure. Little equipment, other than good walking shoes, is needed, and it can be done in segments: a brisk walk after lunch, climbing several flights of stairs instead of using an elevator or escalator, walking instead of driving to the post office. Its benefits are cumulative.

Shoes women wear have caused many to forget how to walk correctly. The knees and ankles should be kept limber, the toes pointed straight ahead. The head should be held high, and the legs should be swung directly ahead, from the hips not from side to side. Shoulders and arms should swing freely and easily. Excessive use of high-heeled shoes makes this stride difficult. It also can cause shortening of the calf muscles and muscles at the back of the thighs, making it uncomfortable to wear low heels and to walk for any period of time.

A walking shoe should have a wide, flat heel; broad, rounded toe; ample room for the toes; a tongue or scree guard to keep out dirt and pebbles; and a rubber sole and heel to absorb impact. "Fit is paramount, no matter what you buy," Dr. Pamilla points out. "The toe caps should be deep enough to let your toes move freely without rubbing. The shoes should be long enough to allow your feet to expand without letting them slide forward when walking downhill. They should be wide enough not to be constrictive, still not permitting your heel to move around while walking."

If you plan to do most of your walking en route to work, your dress shoes can be carried in a small, unobtrusive bag.

Clothing should be lightweight and comfortable, not binding. Try not to overdress during cold weather. Walking burns calories, and as you swing along, you will find yourself warming up. To avoid perspiring and the danger of chilling, you should be able to take off one layer of clothing. Or you can dress to be cool—not cold—when leaving home, and depend on activity to keep you comfortable.

Walking to Adventure

"Hiking the Shenandoahs is an adventure," says Patty R. Royston of Springfield, Virginia. "Every outing offers new experiences, new discoveries. I feel that is why so many of us hike the same areas regularly. There always is change.

"While we are busy in our offices during the week, nature also is working. A tree falls, a trail is diverted, a new flower pokes up. Change is everywhere. I remember trudging along with a group when those up front started 'sshing' us. When I got to the spot where the sshing began, there was an owl sleeping on a tree branch. That was a totally new outdoors experience for me, something I'll never forget—and haven't seen again."

Every year, with other dedicated walkers in the District of Columbia area, Mrs. Royston joins the Level Walkers on their hike along the Chesapeake & Ohio Canal. That tradition was born in 1954 when Supreme Court Justice William O. Douglas led a 180-mile hike of the entire length of the canal, from Cumberland, Maryland, to Washington in a fight to stay the building of a scenic parkway along the route.

Ever since she lived on the side of a mountain in northern Vermont, Carol Nichols, a member of the Overseas Press Club of America, has been a devotee of the Long Trail, one of the nation's most interesting hiking trails. About four years ago she discovered the High Uinta Primitive Area in Utah. The mountain range is unique in that it runs from east to west instead of north to south. "I try to get back there at least once every three years. Backpacking in the wilderness makes me feel as though I am hand in hand with primitive nature. That is a feeling I never have on the Long Trail."

Despite her love for the wilderness, Mrs. Nichols enjoys city hiking, especially in Boston and New York. "I get a thrill wandering side streets and out of the way corners of cities. In the mountains, I cut myself off from my surroundings and become more aware of my body and its responses to the hike. It is almost as though I am encased in a sheath of glass from which I do not emerge until we pitch tent.

"I find almost everyone is quiet for different reasons on the Long Trail. In the city, there is a lot of oohing and aahing among walkers. The experience is different, but still delightful."

Happily for those of us who enjoy moving our bodies, ours is a nation of paths and walks just meant for hiking. And the legions of city walkers who do not long for the rustle of leaves or the crack of branches can find challenge of a different order just around the corner, or a bus or subway ride away.

In Boston, there are walking tours that include Simmons College, the first woman's college in the United States to combine liberal arts and professional education, and the Isabella Stewart Gardner Museum, the home of that noted patron of the arts.

Chicago's lake front offers superb walking paths and vistas of Lake Michigan. Farther west, Denver's parks offer beautifully kept acres for walking. Overlooking the Pacific, San Francisco's Golden Gate area attracts walkers by the scores, while the city itself offers an exciting Chinatown to explore and hills to "lean against" while climbing them.

But most hikers long for the country. By shanks' mare you can walk sections of the Pacific Crest Trail, which runs some 2,350 miles from the Canadian to the Mexican border; the Coronado Trail, which touches on the historic route Francisco de Coronado followed while searching for the fabled Seven Cities of Cibola; or the Apache Trail, which skirts the famed Superstition Mountains as it winds its way from Fish Creek Canyon, Apache and Roosevelt Lakes and ends at Globe, Arizona.

Other western hiking trails include the routes blazed by Lewis and Clark from St. Louis to the mouth of the Columbia River, and the western lore-filled Santa Fe Trail. Unfortunately, many of these areas are now concrete highways, but parallel paths and side roads still are there for the hiking.

Despite the macadamizing of America, there are areas from which all types of motorized vehicles are banned. The famous Appalachian Trail runs the length of the mountain range from Maine to Georgia, touching all but two of the thirteen original colonies. That hike must be done on foot. On the paths leading up to the Appalachian Trail are signs warning casual hikers not to walk the trail unless they are in condition. Although eroded by the ages and not as high or as impressive as the younger Rockies, the Appalachians still are demanding of hikers and are known for their changeable weather. Anyone walking the range must be prepared for sudden rain, wind, and temperature drops.

Perhaps the ultimate hiking experiences are in the nation's Wildernesses and Primitive Areas. Fewer in number than the National Parks and concentrated primarily in the West, they contain secluded areas where the quiet is broken only by the roar of white water or falls, the snap of branches, the rustle of game. When you go in, you go by foot, canoe, or horse. No trail bikes, four-wheel drives, runabouts, or recreation vehicles that can spook game or tear up vulnerable terrain are allowed. You pack in what you need. Unlike the National Parks or their usually nearby state recreation areas, the National Wildernesses have no general stores, no trading posts, no souvenir stands, no neon lights, no lodges. If you have the stamina and the companions—many Rangers suggest that a group should have at least three persons—you can find solitude: a chance to sit by rushing streams and not be bothered by the blare of nearby transistor radios, or to watch wild birds soaring overhead and game climbing cliffs without being distracted by the blare of horns or noise of revving motors.

If you prefer hiking in more "civilized" wildernesses, you have the entire country at your doorstep. No matter where you live, there is likely to be a National Park within a day's drive from your home. Over 30.5 million acres and more than 29,000 developed campsites are included in our National Park system which touches every state of the Union as well as Puerto Rico and the Virgin Islands. Included in the system are seashores, mountains, deserts, lakes, and islands, all set aside for hiking, nature walks, camping, and fishing. And if any facility is overcrowded, the chances are that a few miles down the road there is a state recreational area offering much the same range of facilities.

Apart from a spell of good weather, most important to hiking is a pair of well-fitting, comfortable shoes. For simple city or country walking, even tennis shoes if they have built-in arch supports may be adequate. Once you start walking through forests or up mountain trails, you'll need shoes that protect as well as support your feet.

For day hikes, lightweight trail shoes are more than adequate. They usually are made with a firm cap to prevent toe injuries. They can be waterproofed, and many have scree guards to keep the dirt out. Should you anticipate graduating to backpacking, you should have a heavier pair of boots that will support your weight when loaded down with a pack.

No matter what the advertisements promise, you should break in any new pair of shoes by wearing them evenings and weekends before hiking. There is nothing more depressing while you are on the trail than a blister or a sore spot on your foot from a poorly fitted shoe or one that is still stiff.

You might be able to borrow or rent equipment until you decide on the kind of pack, tent, and other gear you are happy with. Then buy with restraint. Many newcomers to the sport overbuy, accumulating gear that may have looked good in the store but is completely unnecessary on the hike.

There are a number of public membership groups made up of dedicated outdoorspersons. They help maintain many of our hiking trails and, through regional clubs and associations, organize hiking seminars and trips. They include:

The Appalachian Trail Conference
P.O. Box 236
Harpers Ferry, West Virginia 25425

Sierra Club
220 Bush Street
San Francisco, California 94104

Wilderness Society
729 15th Street, NW
Washington, D.C. 20005

For information about state facilities, write to the various states' departments of tourism at the state capitals. For information about federal facilities, write to:

U.S. Department of Agriculture, Forest Service
Washington, D.C. 20250

U.S. Department of the Interior,
Bureau of Sport Fisheries and Wildlife
Washington, D.C. 20240

U.S. Department of the Interior, National Park Service
Washington, D.C. 20240

RACE WALKING

A sport that was extremely popular before it was overshadowed by running is race walking. Happily, the traditional heel-and-toe movement is being seen again.

The gait looks ungainly, but when the legs and arms are accustomed to it, it is comfortable and can eat up the miles without difficulty. The rules state that race walking is a progression of steps so taken that unbroken contact with the ground is maintained, and in particular that, during the period in which a foot is on the ground, the leg shall be straightened (not bent at the knee) at least for one moment.

If you would rather race walk than run, a call to your local Y, Road Runners Club, or newspaper sports desk should put you in touch with other walkers with whom you can work out.

ORIENTEERING

After it was realized that cars could be used for more than just transportation, rallying became a popular sport. Entire families take part in rallies, events that demand the utmost concentration in navigation and precise driving so that teams arrive on schedule at checkpoints, or markers where instructions for the following leg of the course are posted. At times, instructions given the teams are scrambled or written in crossword puzzle form. Cars are penalized for covering the legs too quickly or too slowly.

Leave your car at home. Carry a compass and topographical map instead of a speedometer and odometer. You are orienteering.

Orienteering demands excellent physical conditioning and the ability to use map and compass to select the best possible route between checkpoints. If you are able to read a topographical map and see contour lines as actual terrain in your mind's eye, you can orienteer. If not, the skills can be readily mastered, initially in the comfort of your home and later in easy meets run by orienteering clubs. As you learn, you progress from the simpler meets to the more complicated where you work at night or from map memory only.

Orienteering for Sport and Pleasure by Hans Bengtsson and George Atkinson is an excellent primer, and *Be Expert with Map and Compass* by Björn Kjellström takes the mystery out of that arcane skill. The United States Orienteering Federation, P.O. Box 1039, Ballwin, Missouri 63011, and the Canadian Orienteering Federation, 333 River Road, Vanier, Ontario, have local club addresses and information about the sport.

JOGGING AND RUNNING

Jogging and running are unique among active sports. Unless you are in competition, it really does not matter how good or bad you are. You still can enjoy and gain benefits from them.

You may be an internationally rated Kim Merritt, Jacqueline Hansen, or Miki Gorman who marathon in the 2:30's; hotel chain representative Christiane Dickinson, who was kept out of the 1978 New York Marathon by a pulled tendon; Monaco tourism promotion specialist Maguy Maccario, who runs with Mrs. Dickinson and has just worked up to 8-mile-long runs; airline executive Jessica Morris, who shuttles between bike riding, tennis, and jogging; no matter what, there is a place for you on the running paths. And if you too want to marathon or take part in a group fun run, all you need do is lay down your entry fee if there is one.

The informality of the sport has attracted women by the thousands. There really are no firm numbers as to how many women and men jog regularly. The President's Council on Physical Fitness and Sports estimates there are some 11 million persons who huff and puff on a regular basis. Other estimates put that figure as high as 25 million.

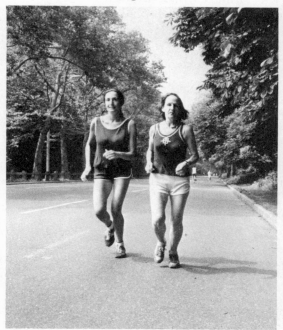

Christiane Dickinson and Maguy Maccario working out for endurance.
(*Jack Galub photo*)

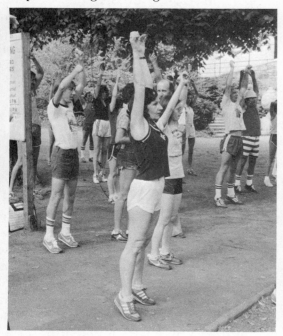

Christiane Dickinson (center) and other runners do stretching exercises before running in weekly session sponsored by New York Road Runners Club.
(*Jack Galub photo*)

There are other indications of the sport's soaring popularity. Whereas once there were only one or two publications for runners, now there are *The Runner, Running Times, Runner's World,* and others. There is scarcely an issue of a popular women's magazine that does not include articles on some aspect of jogging and training.

In 1973, only 395 runners, including 12 women, entered the New York Marathon. That race was held in Central Park, and runners were forced to dodge bicyclists, strollers, and occasional dogs as they covered the 26-mile 385-yard course. By 1977 the New York run had graduated to the streets of the city along a route that touched each of the five boroughs. Among the more than 4,244 entrants were more than 260 women. That field was more than doubled in 1978 to over 11,000 starters of whom more than 1,000 were women. An English school teacher from Oslo, Greta Waitz led the women in the world record time of 2:32:30.

Many women find the mini-marathons more appealing than the grueling long-distance race. In 1972, the first of the annual L'Eggs Mini (10,000 meters) Marathons in the city drew 78 women. That run was won by California's Jacqueline Dixon in 37:01.7. The number of entrants increased gradually each year and in 1976, 492 women entered. Julie Shea of North Carolina won the race in 35:04.8. The 1977 run attracted 2,277 women. It was won by Peg Neppel of Iowa in 34:15.3.

There are a number of sound reasons for this upsurge in running. The sport generally is recognized as a highly efficient means of building cardiovascular fitness, if done on a controlled basis. It has an addictive quality. Perhaps it is the heavier than normal respiration that causes the joy and almost meditative quality running offers that make it difficult to give up the sport once begun.

There are psychological and social factors too. For some, just rounding into shape which permits them to jog at least a mile without stopping is a socially approved, worthwhile personal achievement. They do not want to let go—and why should they? The people who run invariably prove pleasant and companionable. Friendships are begun that hold sway on the running paths only, or may carry over into the runners' mainstream of life. Equipment needed is limited: a good pair of shoes, togs, warm-up suit, or sweat suit are all that is needed. People do not have to reserve time on the running paths as they do on the tennis courts, nor do they have to wait for partners to run with. Invariably, if you wish, there is someone to talk with while running. If not, nobody minds if you work alone.

How to Jog

As in almost any sport, there is correct form. Correct form should be considered as guidelines that help your performance. If yours does not match the consensus offered here, there is no point in being concerned if you are comfortable while running.

Correct jogging form calls for running in an upright, but not stiff position. Your head should be kept up; do not look down at your feet. The arms should be held slightly away from the body, with elbow bent so the forearms are parallel to the ground.

Keep loose while running. If you find you are beginning to stiffen, occasional shaking of the arms and shoulders will help relax you. Taking several deep breaths and blowing them out completely also will help. Otherwise breathe in and out with your mouth open.

There have been various systems of breathing suggested by different physiologists—breathing in on the third step and out on the third after that, for instance—but the chances are you will do well breathing normally. As your heart speeds up, you body will automatically increase your breathing rate.

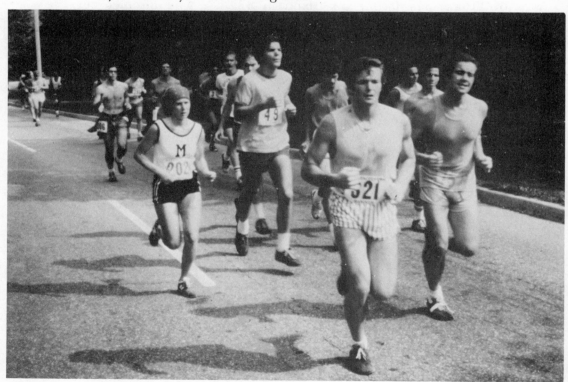

Women today run against men in marathons. (*Jack Galub photo*)

As a youngster in gym class, you probably sprinted, hitting the floor with the balls of the feet. In longer distance running, this style can lead to severe leg soreness. Instead, land on the heel of the foot without thumping and rock the foot forward so you drive off the ball of the foot for your next step. If this is difficult, try a more flat-footed style.

Keep steps short without shuffling, letting your foot hit the ground beneath the knee instead of reaching forward. Do not worry about kicking back or raising your knees high. Leave those styles to sprinters and football backs.

The Difference Between Jogging and Running

There has been considerable discussion of this subtle question. Much of it was sparked by Joe Henderson when he was editor of *Runner's World*. Apart from the semantic satisfactions involved, the dividing line appears to be one of speed. If you are moving at less than 6 miles per hour, you are jogging; over 6, you are running. Otherwise there are few if any substantial differences. Some runners just do not like to be known as joggers. Others do not care as long as they are able to train regularly.

What to Wear

At one time, only track teams dazzled in multi-hued warm-up and running suits. That has changed today. Track suits and warm-ups worthy of Olympic teams now are seen regularly on the jogging paths. In addition to being attractive, they provide a psychological edge that is impossible to have when wearing old-fashioned baggy gray warm-ups.

Clothing that is tight, restricts freedom of movement, or impedes the flow of blood from the legs to the torso should be avoided. Rubberized and plastic suits which are sold to speed weight loss can prove harmful. The increased sweating they produce does not cause permanent weight loss, but does cause body temperature to climb to dangerous levels by interfering with the body's evaporation of sweat. If body moisture cannot evaporate, heatstroke or heat exhaustion may follow.

The freedom running gives should not be a reason for shedding bras. They are needed to avoid tissue injury. Bras should not be tight; they should fit comfortably. If there is nipple irritation from rubbing against the fabric while running, a dab of petroleum jelly will give needed protection.

Some manufacturers now are marketing bras designed especially for runners. They are available in stores catering to runners as well as in some department stores.

Shoes

For years, no more than three or four shoe companies dominated the running market. Now there are many times that number turning out lines of various priced shoes ranging in cost from the low twenties to the high thirties and more.

Women's shoes were an afterthought in the early days of running, and many women either wore small men's sizes or did without. The emergence of women as a dominant force in fitness has caused several makers to change course. Some have added lines made expressly for the female runner, but it still is difficult to find shoes that fit an extremely narrow foot.

Perhaps the best roundup of what shoes are on the market, and what to look for when comparing one brand with another, is the annual shoe issue published in the fall by *Runner's World* magazine. (Bearing in mind, however, that the highest priced shoes—those that the rated runners wear—are not necessarily the best for you.)

The perfect shoe—if there is one—should be:

- Flexible. The shoe should flex easily to avoid unnecessary stress on the foot while running.
- Spacious at the toes. A toe box that offers little room can cause rubbing and chafing of the skin.
- Well cushioned at the heel and throughout the sole, particularly if you are forced to run on hard surfaces or are a beginner. Bypass the thin, minimum-cushioned shoes until you are ready to race and want to sacrifice protection for lightness.
- Supportive. Your arch and heel should be given firm support and cupping.
- Well-made. Rub your hand around the inside of both shoes to make certain there are no rough spots that will prove uncomfortable when running.

And, of course, your shoes must fit well. If you face a choice between a slightly smaller and slightly larger shoe, pick the larger one. Your feet will tend to expand while running and the additional space may be just what you need.

A number of new shoes now feature extra-wide flared heels. These are meant to help prevent knee problems. However, some runners have found they are mixed blessings, helping to cause or aggravate problems. Unless you know from experience that your knees may bother you, buy standard shoes and then take care of them to prevent wearing down.

Before taking a new pair of shoes out to the track, spread a very thin coating of liquified rubber (tubes are sold in many hardware stores) or one of the special preparations sold in athletic shops on the heels where you usually wear them down. Let dry overnight. Then when you run, you will be wearing down the coating instead of the shoe rubber. The life of your heels can be lengthened for many months this way.

WHERE TO RUN

The surfaces you run on should be smooth, be even, and help cushion the impact of your feet on them. Even though our most prestigious marathons are run on highways and roads, for pain-free training you should work on dirt, grass, or boards. Keep pavement for those times when you have no alternative or are preparing for a road race.

PRECEPTS FOR COMPETITION

Sooner or later many joggers feel the urge to compete. Some approach competition as semi-social events. They do not expect to win: they want to complete the course and to enjoy the experience. Others are deadly serious. They want to win or set new personal best times.

Women who compete regularly are willing to give advice freely. They should be listened to because they have paid their dues. Among the group whose suggestions are distilled here are competitors who race regularly and successfully.

- Every race demands training and conditioning. If you have your eyes fixed on an upcoming 6-mile event, make certain you can handle at least 8 miles at speed. Overdistance work will give your body reserves to draw on.
- Train reasonably, emphasizing quality. It is concentration, not socialization, that will give you the stamina you need, but be careful not to overtrain or to overstress your body.

- Get experience and learn to pace yourself by first taking part in informal club meets before entering scheduled races.
- If you want to run, look for meets with small starting fields, often difficult to find in some metropolitan areas. If you must start in the pack, try to move to the side and let the others fight it out. Soon the group will spread out. If you have the speed and conditioning, move up gradually.
- Do not sprint at the start of distance runs. In their eagerness to do well, beginners often start too quickly. They run out of steam and do not finish or else hurt themselves.
- If you do not know the course, cover it the day before the race. Then you will know where the hills are and how far you still have to go at any point.
- Warm up before the race; talk to yourself, if necessary, to remind yourself to keep loose.
- Make certain you are comfortably and sensibly dressed and wear shoes that have been broken in. Remember to double-tie your shoelaces before you start.
- Have a light breakfast of grain cereals, and don't eat until after the race. An apple an hour or so before the event will help peak your energy levels.
- Make certain you visit the rest room at least one-half hour before starting time.
- Take all water stops. If you are accustomed to drinking water rather than commercial drinks, do not switch during the race. You may upset your stomach. Similarly, do not experiment with new diets or foods during the few days before the meet.
- If you can, cover the course in the shade out of the sun. Do not allow yourself to become overheated or dehydrated. Avoid exhaustion.
- Ask friends or family to time you at specified distances so you will know how fast you are running. Your personal after-race analysis will help you pace yourself better in your next runs.
- Set reasonable goals for yourself, especially during your first runs. You want to walk off content that you have finished the distance and have done well.

Whether to wear socks is the only question about which there appears substantial disagreement. A number of people wear them to help absorb impact. Some wear an extremely thin sock under the bulky gym sock to protect against chafing, and some wear the shoe-high short sock. Many women wear bulky socks only to keep their shoes fitting correctly. Some do not wear them at all, in order, they say, to avoid being slowed by socks heavy with perspiration. For the beginner, most racers recommend they be worn, at least until she becomes accustomed to competition.

FOR MORE FUN! MIX JOGGING AND EXERCISE

On those days that discourage even the most dedicated fitness addict, don't curl up in front of the TV. Instead run your personal in-home circuit course.

All you need is a modest amount of space, three or four rooms to run through, and perhaps a flight of stairs on which to jog up and down. With that as your cardiovascular foundation, set up stops or stations where you will do specific stretching-flexibility, warm-up, and weight training exercises. Run the course and work out at a fast pace, making certain not to trip over furniture, and you will find yourself working nearly as hard as you would outdoors.

There is no need to keep your in-home circuit indoors. The Denver YMCA took a similar course and expanded it into the 1½-mile-long Washington Park Life Fitness Trail. If you follow the instructions on placards at each station, you find yourself doing progressively more vigorous exercises. Afterward you might taper off with one easy nonstop loop of the circuit if you have endurance needed at that mile-high altitude.

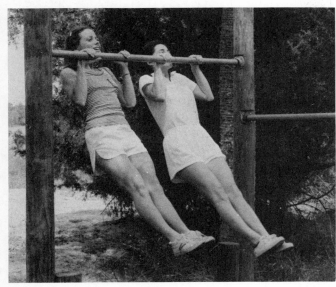

Doing pull-ups to strengthen the upper body on the Fripp Island Parcourse.
(Fripp Island photo)

A more demanding workout is offered by the Parcourse, a circuit that traces its roots to Europe. As set up at Fripp Island, a South Carolina residential community, the 1½-mile course includes eighteen exercise stations. You walk the first five stations for warm-up, and then jog the remainder. The exercises call for jumping jacks, touch-stretches, hop kicks, knee lifts, step-ups, circle body on overhead rings, isometric squats, chin-ups, vault bars, toe touches, sit-ups, body curls on a slant board, push-ups, bench leg-raises, hand walks on parallel bars, leg stretches and, finally, balance beam walks.

There now are more than 100 mini- and full-length Parcourses scattered across the country in parks, schools, universities, Y's, and hotels. Try one the next time you are traveling. They're a nonalcoholic pick-me-up.

RUNNING OBSTACLES FOR TIME

Parcourses and Life Fitness Trails are outgrowths of the military obstacle course, which is planned not for torture, but to exercise every muscle in the body, to help develop coordination and confidence.

Invariably trainees approach the course with horror and dread. After the first few times around, as mind and body learn to work together to cut obstacles down to size, the course becomes more fun than challenge. Then they start racing the clock, outdoing their previous times.

The Academy's obstacle course is only 870 yards long, 10 yards short of a half-mile. But its fourteen obstacles are designed to exercise every part of the body, to make every muscle do the job it was created for. If you were an observer, you would, for instance, watch the women cadets race to the water jump, pushing off as they grasp a rope. Those holding on too long find themselves back over the water ditch. Those who let go too quickly also find themselves in the water. But up they come, soggy and muddy, running for the hurdles and the finish. Soon they march off looking as though they had done nothing more than taken part in a vigorous exercise class.

It looks like a real workout, and it is, but remember that hundreds of women have turned that tiger of a course into a pussycat. Given the training and conditioning, you probably would too.

Let us run the obstacle course here, just to see the challenge many of the women cadets faced for the first time in their lives—and overcame.

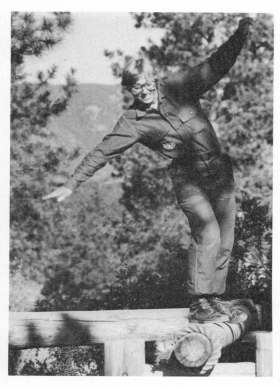

The rolling log tests balance as cadets run the obstacle or confidence course.

A cadet weaves her way over one of the obstacles that exercise each part of her body as she covers the obstacle course.

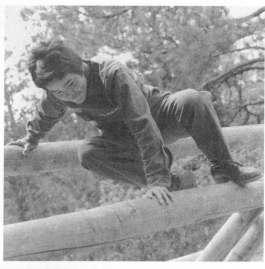

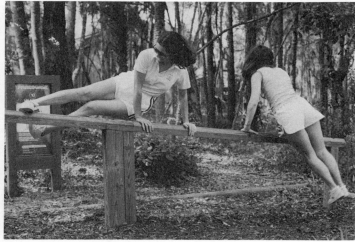

Swinging to build coordination and agility on the Fripp Island course. *(Fripp Island photo)*

Obstacle 1. Log Balance: You approach the logs at a full run. You pick one and walk over it as quickly as possible. If you fall into the water, you wade to the other side of the ditch. If you fall on the log, you stand up and start moving again.

Obstacle 2. Vault and Roll: These obstacles are a series of five horizontal logs. Again, you come in at a run, place both hands on the first log and swing your body over. At the second, you throw your body to the ground and roll under. You follow that same over and under vault and roll until you have done all five. Then you start running toward the ladder barrier.

Obstacle 3. Ladder Barrier: The ladder barrier has two cargo nets, one to climb up and the other to climb down. Going up the ladder, you should hold your body close to the net and keep your eyes raised to the top. On reaching the platform on top, you crawl across it and then go down the other side the same way. You must stay on the rope ladder until both feet are on the ground; jumping is not allowed.

Obstacle 4. Handrail: At first glance, this looks easy, but it is one of the most difficult course obstacles so far as upper body strength is concerned, and many cadets just can't make it at first. You grab onto two parallel rails, raise yourself into the air and shuffle or "walk" the length of the bar with your hands on the rail. Feet must not touch the ground while you are on the handrails. If they do, you start over. Many cadets do.

Obstacle 5. Belly Under: You belly under, crawling through one obstacle to a log pile, roll over the pile and creep through a second obstacle. Cadets who have been trapped under the barrier have been known to dig their way out with their hands.

Obstacle 6. Wall Climb and Log Balance: Climb the wall, and cross the balance beams beyond as quickly as possible.

Obstacle 7. High Step-Over: There are fifteen ropes strung about two feet above the group between parallel bars. Each rope must be stepped over, alternating the lead foot. It is suggested you step over one rope at a time to avoid the danger of falling. Stepping on the ropes is forbidden.

Obstacle 8. Horizontal Ladder: You have seen this one in your gym class but may not have had the chance to try it. You jump up and grab the crossbars and start swinging, hand over hand, to the end of the ladder. You may skip as many of the crossbars as you can, but you must swing from the first and last crossbar. The odds are that you will fall if you try to do the ladder too rapidly to get it over with.

Obstacle 9. Water Jump: You run and jump over a water-filled ditch, landing with both feet on the ground at the same time. Your knees should be flexed to absorb the impact and your body should be inclined slightly forward.

Obstacle 10. Opossum Hang: Opossums do it more easily. You grab the horizontal bar with both arms and legs, and as you hang below it you propel yourself along the bar until your feet touch the down-course vertical support.

Obstacle 11. Balance Beams: Three horizontal bars are placed end to end in a zigzag. You leap onto the top of one of the beams and cover the Z. You should take this obstacle as quickly as you can—without falling off.

Obstacle 12. Horizontal Triangle: Five bars are mounted on a horizontal triangle, two on each side below the apex. You jump up on the first bar and go over it, under the second, over the third or top bar, under the fourth bar, and over the fifth.

Obstacle 13. The Water Swing: You run up toward the hanging ropes, grab one, holding both hands close together, and pull forward. Near the top of your arc, thrust your legs forward and let go of the rope. Your momentum should carry you beyond the ditch. If you let go too soon or too late, you fall in the water below.

Obstacle 14. Four Log Hurdles: These are to be jumped in any manner you wish. But you may not run around or climb under them. Then you sprint some 200 yards to the finish line.

Congratulations! You've just covered the Academy obstacle course.

Other Sports
You Can Enjoy

There are a variety of individual and team sports in which you can take part and even reach competitive levels as do the women cadets. Blended into your total fitness program, they provide a stimulating change of activity, help avoid sameness, train your muscles in new skills, and broaden your friendships.

Only a few of these sports will be covered here to illustrate the many from which you may choose. The Academy coaching memorandums in Chapter 5 point the way to most of those.

The demands placed on your body and cardiovascular system by each depend on the vigor with which you play. A game of tennis doubles, for instance, does not force you to work as hard as singles. Horseback riding will not increase your heartbeat as rapidly as a long-distance run.

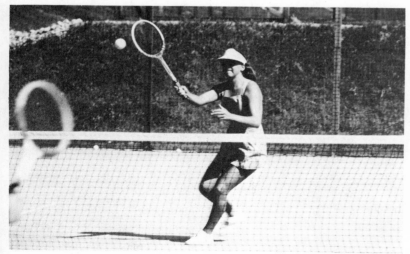

Videotape recordings, ball machine teaching lanes, expert coaches combine to instruct women in tennis at Killington Ski Resort in central Vermont. Women are becoming increasingly significant in professional and amateur tennis. *(Bob Perry photo)*

For some activities, such as mountain climbing, tennis, and gymnastics, you should have coaching. Tennis elbows are not foreign to women who buy racquets that are too heavy or who do not handle their racquets correctly. In mountain climbing, incorrect techniques used on the face of a steep rise can be disastrous.

BICYCLING*

The two-wheel bicycle is an elegant form of natural transportation. Its wheels and assorted gears are designed to translate foot power into motion with a minimum of energy waste. They are built to meet different age groups' needs. There are tricycles for youngsters, two wheels for teenagers and adults, and again three-wheel bicycles for older persons who worry about possible spills.

The resurgence of interest in bike riding in the 1960's was due in part to medical opinion that it is an excellent antidote for lazy cardiovascular systems. The late Dr. Paul Dudley White, the noted heart specialist, was emphatic in prescribing riding as a good way to "prevent heart disease." It also helps control weight, burning up between 300 and 600 calories an hour, if you restrain the urge to coast and to use your low gears on hills.

Biking is recognized as one of the four "best exercises," along with walking, jogging, and swimming. But bikes have one unequaled advantage: on wheels you cover a lot more ground, so the bicycle is a practical means of transportation—and, just as important to many, it is nonpolluting and does not use up natural resources. Bicycling also is one of the few outdoor sports in which almost nobody is too young or too old to take part.

Learning to Ride: If you cycled as a youngster, you may wobble a bit at first, but you'll quickly be rolling. If you are a beginner, you probably will need a few lessons.

The basic principle underlying riding is right out of the physics texts. Stand a coin on edge and it falls over. Roll it and it stays up. The theory applies to riding: If you are moving, you won't fall. So much for theory. Reality is a bit different. You can tip over until you learn to balance and control the bike.

It usually is easier to learn on women's models: they are easier to get on and off. At first, keep the saddle and handlebars as low as possible. Sit on the bike and push it along, raising your feet every so often and letting it coast. Once you have learned to coast, you start using the pedals. A friend may hold the bike lightly until you learn to pedal easily.

With few exceptions, geared adult bikes are equipped with front and rear wheel caliper brakes. Squeezing on the handlebar brake levers causes the calipers to move together, pressing the brake pads against the wheels' metal rims. This brake action is simple and efficient, but remember to use the rear brakes before the front or you may be flipped over the handlebars. Use a rapid pressure-release-pressure action rather than a steady squeeze which tends to glaze the brake pads and make them ineffective.

The brakes on three-speed bikes are hidden within the axle of the rear wheel. To stop, you back-pedal, applying pressure to the brakes until the bike stops.

As you gain confidence, begin raising the saddle and handlebars. Good riding depends on getting the maximum power from your leg muscles. This calls for a seat high enough to let you extend your leg during the down or power thrust. Your ankles can then swivel easily for the bottoming and up push. You will find it a lot easier and more efficient to use the balls of your feet on the pedals rather than the instep or heel. Knees should be pointed straight ahead.

The saddle should be kept horizontal at first, with the tip directly above the center of the pedal wheel or two inches or so to the rear. Later, you may find a down or up tilt of the seat more comfortable.

Handlebars should be about level with the seat. Raising them slightly higher is sometimes more comfortable for women, but too much of a rise makes the bike harder to control.

Learning About Gears: Learning to use your bike's gears or speeds is the last step in becoming a good rider.

As in the pre-automatic transmission cars, low gears are there to help you conquer hills with a minimum of effort, unless you are riding for cardiovascular enhancement.

The typical rented bike is a three-speed. Learning to use its gears presents little problem. As you reach a hill, ease up on the pedals and move the shift key. On some three-speeds you may have to back-pedal slightly during the shift.

Some adult bikes have five-speed or ten-speed gears. These are somewhat harder to handle. At first have the dealer work the gears in the store. He usually does this by hanging the bike from the ceiling and then turning the pedals by hand. At home, turn the bike upside down or prop the rear wheel between two chairs and shift while turning the pedals. If you shift while the wheels are not turning, you may ruin the shift transport.

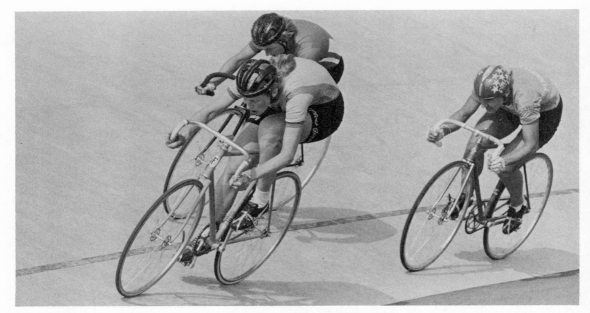

Five-time national champion Connie Carpenter drives past Nancy Kaiser and Mary Jane Roech to win at the Trexlertown Velodrome near Allentown, Pennsylvania. (*John Chay photo*)

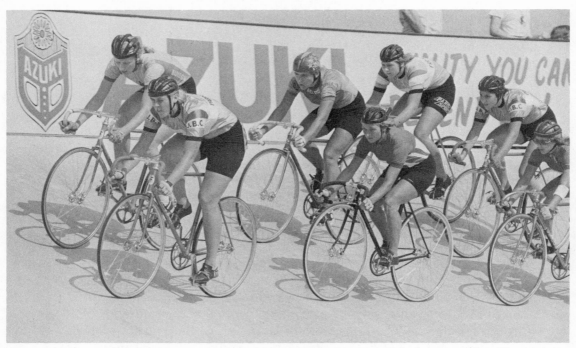

Women riders train and compete regularly at the Trexlertown Velodrome. (*John Chay photo*)

For the average rider, a gear ratio in the 60's is normal. Anything over 70 is considered high and under 60 is low. A racing bicycle's range covers 55 to 100 or more. Touring bikes offer a good range of low gears, in the 30's and up. A five-speed can range from close to 34 to as high as 88, and a three-speed from around 50 up to 90. Your bicycle store mechanic can help you select the gear ratios best for your riding needs.

There are almost as many bikes on the market as automobiles. They are built by American companies, and imported from Britain, France, India, Canada, Japan, and Italy. Selection of the type and model depends on the kind of riding you plan to do, your budget, and storage space.

The Coaster: These are built for hard, minimum-care use. They have wide saddles, rugged balloon tires, coaster brakes, and heavy fenders. They also have two major drawbacks. They do not have gears and they weigh about 40 pounds. Coasters are excellent for short-distance utility use—shopping, visiting, picnicking, and exercise.

The Three-Speed: This is the standard bike for most adults. The three-speeds help on hills. They can be used for carrying light loads in a front basket or on a rear fender. They are lighter than the coasters but not overly sensitive to various conditions.

The Five-Speed and Ten-Speed: The five-speed and particularly the ten-speed bikes are built for serious riding: touring, hosteling, vacation, and commuting. Although their narrow saddles take some breaking in, they are the most comfortable for long-distance riding. They often have turned-under handlebars that make it possible to change hand positions, and metal pedals that are easier to use in wet weather.

Bike Touring: Touring is an excellent means of visiting new places while building stamina. The easiest way to prepare for longer trips is to take short ones regularly, and then gradually lengthen the time you spend on your bicycle. If you can ride three times a week, begin with at least 4 miles. At a healthy clip, this will take you less than 30 minutes. (Most good riders average between 10 and 12 miles per hour.) Don't dally on these trips. Instead speed up every so often. This will teach you to ride fast in addition to building stamina. Soon you will be able to increase the distance you travel to 5, 6, 7, and 8 miles. On all trips, stop every hour for ten minutes to munch raisins or just walk around.

Bicycle touring is simple, particularly now that communities in every part of the country have marked bike trails to help make riding easier and safer. One of the longest trails links Kenosha and LaCrosse, about 320 miles across Wisconsin. Others circle Pikes Peak and touch the Garden of the Gods in Colorado Springs, cover the route taken by the Forty-niners during the California Gold Rush, tour Louisiana's bayou country, and follow the Connecticut River into northern New England.

Bus companies, airlines, and railroads have space for your bike should you decide to start your tour a half continent or more away. Or you can attach your bike to an easily installed car roof or rear bumper bike rack.

There are many advantages to group touring, apart from the friendships that can be made. Often the group takes along a station wagon or minibus for bed rolls and other equipment. You also pick up pointers on correct riding technique, and if something goes wrong with your bike, someone can usually fix it immediately.

If you are interested in touring, the League of American Wheelman, 19 South Bothwell, Palatine, Illinois 60067, and American Youth Hostels, National Campus, Delaplane, Virginia 22025, will put you in touch with local groups.

Increasingly, women now are taking part in bicycle road and track competitions. Recently, a 75-mile race in New York City attracted women riders. The Red Zinger Bicycle Classic in which women take part is regarded as one of the best road competitions in the country, and the Bicycling International Madison Championship sponsored by *Bicycling* magazine and held at The Trexlertown Velodrome near Allentown, Pennsylvania, attracts an international group of riders. Your local bicycle shop can open the door for you to club racing if you care to pursue the sport.

SWIMMING

Terry Wood LaVine, an international oil company executive, is one of the fortunate ones. There is a swimming pool in her apartment house, and six evenings a week find her and her husband doing laps and exercises. The workouts keep them trim and physically fit.

Most women are born to swim. They have greater buoyancy than men, and in many ways noncompetitive swimming is gentler to the body than jogging or gymnastics. There is none of the jar of the body on the dismount in gymnastics or the foot impact of jogging that may cause knee and tendon injuries.

It is a pity that so few persons have easy access to swimming facilities, for swimming is a perfect exercise. Done correctly, it exercises the cardiovascular system as well as every muscle of the body.

For pool swimming, the variety of strokes needed is limited: the breast stroke, rudimentary back stroke, and perhaps for occasional bursts of speed, the crawl. Each can be easily learned, and once mastered, they are never forgotten.

Swimming sessions should be preceded by a long hot shower to lessen the danger of musculoskeletal problems. Afterward some five to ten minutes should be spent swimming slowly and doing exercise at poolside to warm up.

Your swimming program should start gradually—four 25-yard swims for the first two weeks, two 100-yard laps for the third to fifth weeks, four 100-yard laps for the sixth to fourteenth weeks, and then building up to a minimum of four 200-yard swims by the end of the thirty-first week.

Laps should be done at a steady, comfortable rate of speed, monitoring your pulse from time to time. The built-in handicap of swimming is the social aspect of the sport. The chance to sit at poolside and chat can prove too much of an attraction at times. Restrain the urge; talk after you have done your laps or during brief rest periods. Finish your workouts with a tepid shower.

An optimum swimming program calls for a workout daily. But for the average swimmer, three or four workouts a week are sufficient, especially if you alternate your sessions with tennis, fast walking, or another sport.

Nonswimmers also can use pools for exercise. The resistance of water to body movement offers the same strengthening effects as does working with weights, without the stress that weight training entails. Walking rapidly or running through waist-high water with palms extended is excellent for hips, stomach, and leg muscles. So is walking rapidly with legs spread apart. Hopping and jumping forward strengthens the lower half of the body.

For maximum pool enjoyment, you should learn to swim if you do not know how. The rudiments can be quickly learned at a Y. Many pools offer instruction, and so do some public schools and local community recreation departments.

SKIING

Few active sports match the exhilaration and satisfaction of Alpine, or as it is often called, downhill skiing, and women by the thousands have responded to the lure of fresh snow on the hills. Singles and marrieds alike often drive all night for a weekend of skiing and then return on a Monday morning tired but content after another long night drive.

As the sport becomes increasingly sophisticated and the slopes more crowded, it is important that correct techniques be mastered and proper equipment used. At the larger ski developments such as Killington in Vermont, ski instruction and outfitting have been developed to a high degree of efficiency. Equipment, if it is needed, is matched to the needs of the beginner as well as the advanced skier, and nonskiers are taught through the use of an Accelerated Ski Method.

This approach uses short skis initially with gradual advancement to longer skis, until the skier eventually uses equipment matched to her height, weight, and ability. "Ground instruction" is as important to the method as actual on-snow work. The novice attends clinics and films and is given an opportunity to discuss her problems with instructors. She also is advised regarding the purchase of boots, skis, and clothing.

Three basic factors are stressed during instruction: control, speed, and terrain. Control enables you to stop at any time you wish and to avoid skiing into other skiers or standing objects. It will also enable you to avoid being hit by someone racing toward you. Experts suggest that you ski conservatively so if you fall, miscalculate, or are forced to change direction suddenly, you can do so without injuring yourself.

The speed at which you choose to ski is directly related to your assessment of snow conditions, traffic, your own skiing ability, the abilities of other skiers, weather, and terrain. The "hot skier" who is not considerate of others can create as much havoc on the slopes as the suddenly out of control novice.

Map trails should be studied carefully. Before going out, know which lifts take you to the trails you can ski safely, and know how to read the National Ski Area Association trail markers. Green circle markers indicate the least difficult trails and slopes, blue squares are more difficult, and black diamonds the most difficult. The ability to ski expertly on one black diamond trail does not guarantee that you can cope with all difficult trails. They vary significantly even within the same area. A rectangle, yellow with a red border, warns that a trail is closed to skiers. A red triangle with a yellow exclamation mark in the

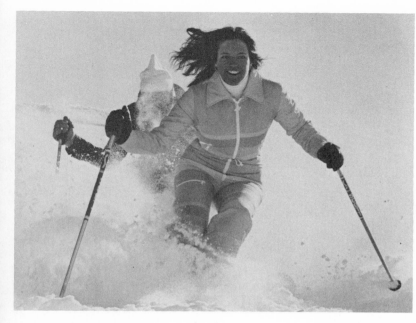

Control as well as speed is stressed at Keystone Mountain, Colorado. *(Keystone Resort photo)*

center is a warning that there are difficult areas or obstacles ahead.

The past few years have seen increasing numbers of skiers who have become tired of the long waits on slopes and have turned to cross-country skiing and ski touring. In cross-country you travel overland on marked routes, and in ski touring you may blaze your own trail. The physical demands of these two sports are about double those of Alpine skiing.

A good level of conditioning is important, and beginners are advised to start slowly until they have accustomed their musculoskeletal and cardiovascular systems to cross-country or ski touring.

Jana Hlavaty first represented Czechoslovakia in international cross-country skiing competition. After she became an American citizen, she won a place on the United States Olympic team. Today, she is cross-country skiing director at Keystone, a Colorado resort.

Mrs. Hlavaty says almost anyone in good health can ski cross-country because "it is a natural movement, like walking, and is physically beneficial; but you must train before you begin." When Mrs. Hlavaty was on the United States teams, competitive cross-country ski training included running during the summer, roller skiing on roads, and weight training. Sessions lasted four to five hours a day, seven days a week.

For the poorly conditioned woman interested in ski travel, she urges that first an exercise stress test be taken, or at least a resting electrocardiogram. Then the warm months should be spent getting into shape before the snows fall.

The training should start with walking followed by jogging: 15 minutes of walking alternating with 5 minutes of jogging, gradually building up to 2 miles of jogging. This, she believes, merely lays the foundation to fitness that includes the ability to run 5 miles at an 8- to 12-minute mile rate, depending on age, at least four times a week.

There are a good range of exercises for strengthening the muscles used in skiing.

1. *Side-to-side jumping:* Stand with feet and knees together, knees bent. Keeping them in that position, jump at least two feet from left to right, and then back again. Each round trip equals one repetition. Beginning with 5 repetitions, then 10, build yourself up gradually to 25 or more repetitions.

2. *Push-ups.* After building yourself up with on-floor push-ups, increase the stress on your arms and shoulders by switching to other more demanding positions. You can either dip while holding onto the backs of two chairs, or place your hands on the seat of a chair while your body is extended in a full-length push-up position. Build up to 10 repetitions if you can.

3. *Squat-sit against wall.* Stand about 10 inches from a wall, and gradually lower your body to a sitting position. When your thighs are parallel to the floor, raise the heels as high as possible. Initially hold for 10 seconds and then gradually work your way up to 15, 20, and eventually 30 seconds. If there is any sharp pain in your knees during this exercise, stop and omit it for several days. If the pain returns while you are exercising, limit the time spent or omit the exercise completely.

4. *Tendon stretch.* Put your hands flat against a wall, face high. Move your feet backward without shifting your hands until your body is straight and your heels barely make contact with the floor. Then push down, setting the heels on the floor. Gradually inch your feet backward until your heels no longer touch the floor. Several repetitions are ample in an exercise session.

5. *Bent-leg sit-up.* Lie on your back. Draw your feet up bending your knees until the angle of your legs to your thighs is about 90°. Clasp your hands behind your head. Curl your back up smoothly raising your trunk until it is vertical to the floor and then ease back down to the starting position. If you do not have a partner who can hold your feet down while you are doing sit-ups, anchor them under a desk, chest, or other heavy piece of furniture. Work your way up to 30 repetitions.

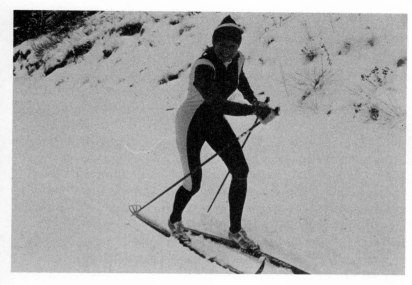

Former Olympian Jana Hlavaty is cross-country skiing director at Keystone Resort, Colorado. (*Keystone Resort photo*)

Cross-country skiing is not as difficult to learn as Alpine, nor is it as expensive. Clothing need not be chic; shoes are inexpensive, but they must fit comfortably; and skis and poles need not be top of the line. At first, you probably can make do with what you have in your wardrobe. Avoid cotton jeans and synthetics. Woolen slacks and sweat socks plus a lightweight woolen sweater and a thin parka will be more than ample. Don't forget a wool knit hat, warm gloves, and sunglasses.

Mrs. Hlavaty advocates layering for warmth. Two or three light layers of clothing are more practical, and safer too, for cross-country skiing or ski touring: a thin glove under a heavier one, a sleeveless down jacket over a sweater instead of bulky parkas, and a thin pair of socks under a slightly heavier pair. When you start overheating, simply peel off a layer of outer clothing and either drape it over a tree branch or tie it around your waist to avoid perspiring.

Rent or borrow equipment until you learn. There is little point in buying until you decide that you and the sport are compatible.

Skis should be chosen to match the terrain. Mountainous areas call for heavier skis than rolling or flat country. Generally speaking, there are two types of skis—heavier general touring skis that you may wear, if you wish, with ordinary hiking boots along with a cable binding around the heel with a safety front throw; and lighter skis that require special boots which fit into a toe clamp, with the heel left free to lift off the ski. Skis should be long enough to reach about four inches below your wrist while you are holding your arm straight up.

Poles should be long enough to tuck under the armpit as you

stand. They should be lightweight with adjustable handstraps so you can switch from light to bulky gloves if necessary.

Cross-country, unlike Alpine, can be learned from a friend or even an illustrated book. Many of the 350,000 devotees of the sport in the United States are self-taught. Later instruction at a school will provide the finer points. In the teach-yourself method, principally you learn to stand, fall, and walk; then to climb a hill, turn, go down the slope, and stop. Emphasis is on control. You learn to fall almost at once because that is what usually happens the first time you stand up on skis. The trick of falling safely is learning simply to sit down. It is almost impossible to hurt yourself this way and you are in a good position for getting back on your feet again.

An invaluable source of information about ski touring and cross-country techniques, equipment, areas, schools, and tours is the Ski Touring Council at West Hill Road, Troy, Vermont 05868, Mr. Rudolf F. Mattesich, president. The group's annual Ski Touring Guide and Ski Touring Schedule should be read by every woman interested in the sport.

FENCING

Douglas Fairbanks, Sr., and Errol Flynn hung from rafters while wielding swords that made them invulnerable to movie foes. Today the fairy princesses they fought for probably would outfence them.

Women make up a large segment of the fencing population. For Priscilla De Marinis, an assistant editor, the sport has a romantic quality. It also has aesthetic appeal. She started four years ago. For two years she fenced once a week at a Y, and then she decided to become more seriously involved with the sport. Today she fences at least twice a week in addition to her weekly lesson at the Santelli School of Fencing in New York City. She also competes in the metropolitan division of the Amateur Fencers League of America. The AFLA, which was established in 1891, governs 60 regional branches, tournaments, and Olympic teams.

Until recently, women fenced only in foil. Now the AFLA has scheduled women's matches in epee and saber as well, a reflection of growing interest among women in competitive fencing.

If fencing has a drawback, it is that it is not a spectator sport, unless the spectator is a fencer. "It is a sport that stresses the minimal motion—a subtle parry enough to deflect the opponent's blade and

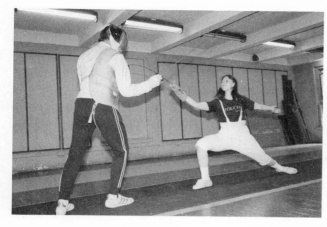

Priscilla De Marinis trains with her coach at the Santelli School of Fencing. *(Jack Galub photo)*

leave the defender in a position to make a riposte or counterthrust," says Miklos Bartha of the Santelli School. Mr. Bartha finds that fencing strips away the psychological armor many of his students wear. After a time, they become more outgoing, more vigorous, and they themselves comment on the changes they go through.

Fencing is not a natural sport. The body must assume specialized positions that are demanded by the advance and retreat, the lunge and recovery, the attack and defense. How the fencer executes her attack depends on her style, skill, and imagination. During lessons and fencing sessions, the fundamental hand and foot movements, the attack, defense, and retreat are practiced until the movements become instinctive. The skilled fencer does not stop to think about what she does next. Conditioned reflexes and instinct take hold. She executes her movements smoothly with the precision and economy of movement needed to protect herself.

If a woman is physically healthy and has a good level of cardiovascular stamina, she can start fencing even in her early sixties. She will be slower than younger women, but in most large groups she will find others about her age to work against.

Serious fencers are expected to keep their cardiovascular stamina at high levels and to do flexibility and warm-up exercises regularly. If you follow the Air Force Academy program, you need only add the specialized exercises required by the demands of the sport. These include:

- *One-leg deep-knee bend:* with right leg extended, bend on left leg. Alternate.
- *Jump and turn:* Jump quarter turn to the right, quarter turn to the left, then half turn to the right, half turn to the left; finally, three-quarter turn to the right, three-quarter turn to the left.

- *Squat jump:* Stand with hands clasped behind head, feet four to six inches apart. Squat on right heel. Jump up with body and legs straight; thrust the rear foot forward while in the air. Squat on left heel and repeat.

Other exercises include standing back bends. Bend back with hands stretched overhead; follow by toe touching, alternate toe touching with legs spread apart, and lunges.

Being able to shine competitively usually takes seven to ten years of hard work. Many women believe the challenge is worthwhile and fence competitively. For others, like Miss De Marinis, the sport itself, the physical conditioning and enjoyment it offers, as well as the friendships that may be made, are satisfaction enough.

Fencing is not particularly expensive. Basic attire—foil, mask, jacket, breast protector, and glove—costs anywhere from $70 to $90. Schools often offer packaged series and single lessons, and will lend equipment free of charge until newcomers decide they like the sport.

CANOEING/KAYAKING

Canoes and kayaks are fun. They are not just an excuse for lazing in the sun; rather they are an open sesame to fast travel that lets you search out nooks and bends in rivers and lake shores you never would know existed if you backpacked or rode past.

Molly Stark, who is special projects editor for *Wilderness Camping* magazine and an avid canoeist, suggests you learn in the stern position of a two-person boat, at least until you get your upper body and stomach muscles ready for the workout. The bow or front is the strength position. Stern paddling mainly keeps the boat on course, a task that does not demand power. As you become familiar with boat handling and your muscles become accustomed to working the paddle, you learn to apply power to your strokes and move up to the bow. From that point on you can learn to handle one-person canoes and kayaks.

An experienced Colorado kayak instructor finds that women often learn to handle kayaks more readily than men. They usually are more comfortable than men in the boats, and once they get over what fear they might have of tipping, they have the potential to become first class kayakers.

The sport appears more difficult than it actually is. Kayaks look fragile, but they have been proved sound by centuries of use in the Arctic and on white water rivers. At first, you learn to handle your twin-blade paddle on dry land, practicing the push stroke, learning to use your shoulders for power. A broomstick can also be used to accustom your muscles to the paddling motion. Then you learn how to get into the kayak, to jiggle the boat with your knees, to turn in either direction, and to tip over. Sooner or later, the chances are you will tip—just as an equestrienne is thrown—you should practice leaving the kayak and recovering.

You will find the chances of hitting your head against a lake bottom are slim, but greater on fast water or white water. Still you should get into the habit of wearing a helmet at all times when kayaking. Either a hockey or special kayaking helmet will do. You should also know how to swim and should wear a Coast Guard-approved Personal Flotation Device (PFD). It is good safety practice to have one on even when out in a broad-beam canoe on a placid lake, and to make certain that all children and anyone else wear theirs. Storms blow up unexpectedly, and even the most stable canoes can be tipped if improperly handled.

Should you become serious about kayaking, you will want to buy a wet suit if you expect to be out on cold water. Otherwise, woolen—not cotton or synthetics—pants, shirt, and a water repellent windbreaker will provide the warmth you need even when wet.

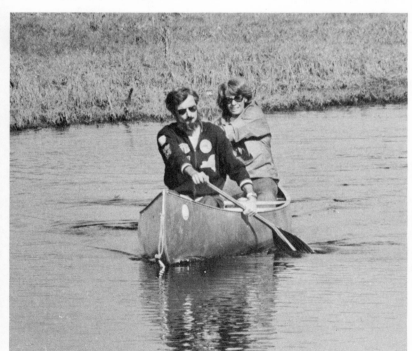

Molly Stark and *Wilderness Camping* editor Harry Roberts demonstrate correct paddling technique. Note the bent paddle, preferred by many experienced canoeists. *(Wilderness Camping photo)*

Canoeing and kayaking demand shoulder and upper arm strength, as well as firm stomach and thigh muscles. The Academy exercises in Chapter 2 include those you should concentrate on: sit-ups, push-ups, body benders. In addition, there is the sitting stretch. Sit on the floor with your legs extended and separated, and with your hands resting on your knees; slowly bend forward, stretching as far forward as you can with your hands.

There are a number of associations and publications covering the sport and club activities. They include The American Canoe Association, 4260 East Evans Avenue, Denver, Colorado 8022; United States Canoe Association, 216 Inverness Drive, Lexington, Kentucky 50503; American Whitewater Affiliation, P.O. Box 1584, San Bruno, California 94066; *Canoe*, 1999 Shepard Road, St. Paul, Minnesota 55116; *Down River*, Box 366, Mountain View, California 94042; and *Wilderness Camping*, 1597 Union Street, Schenectady, New York 12309.

WHY SOME ATHLETES WIN, OTHERS LOSE

Should you take part in competition, you probably will wonder why some athletes outrun, outrace, outswim others who may have worked just as hard and even received the same coaching.

There are a host of tangible and intangible factors that affect winning and losing. There are up and down days. Biorhythms aside, there are just days when you may be nursing a cold that hasn't surfaced or are being affected by family or work tensions. There is also the question of motivation: Are you prepared to make that second and even third effort needed to win?

There also is the reality that some women are better athletes than others. Their reflexes may be sharper. They may be younger. Age doesn't seem to be too much of a factor in long-distance running, though, up to a point, of course. Generally, the mature runner is a better marathoner than the younger, overeager competitor who peaks too soon in the race.

Your physiology plays a major role in whether you lead the field. Our muscles contain both fast and slow twitch fibers. If yours have a preponderance of fast twitch fibers, you probably are a speedster. If your muscles are made up largely of slow twitch fibers, all the effort in the world won't help you set a sprint record.

With the right combination of fibers, you may become a champion miler, marathoner, swimmer, canoeist, distance bicyclist. With hard work and motivation, you may even change your distance and specialty.

Anne Henning successfully transformed herself from a speedster into a strong, all-around athlete. In 1972 she set an Olympic record for the 500=meter speed skating event and then went on to win a bronze in the 1,000 meters. After the Olympics she won two firsts in the ABC Network Superstars sports competition. When I last spoke with her she was running longer distances at Keystone, taking advantage of the high altitude to build stamina.

Another woman who successfully changed her sport is internationally ranked Nina Kuscsik, who regularly is either top woman or among the first women to finish in distance runs. She was among seven women who raced in the 1972 Boston Marathon and was the first of the group to cross the finish line. Five years later she set a new women's American record for 50 miles, doing the distance in 6:35:53. In April 1978 she was the first woman to finish in the 10-kilometer Bloomingdale/Perrier road race. She ran that in 39:21:7, outstanding time for a woman who is nudging 40 years of age. Associated with Mt. Sinai Hospital in New York City, Nina Kuscsik finds the time to train and compete regularly, despite her job and the demands of her private life.

Are you another Henning or Kuscsik? You'll never know until you try. Even if you don't win marathons, you can compete purely for the fun and excitement. Many women do.

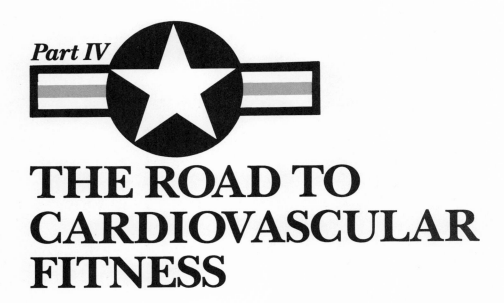

Part IV

THE ROAD TO CARDIOVASCULAR FITNESS

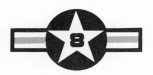

Age Is No Barrier— Time Can Be Made

With increasing regularity, stories appear of women in their seventies and eighties who climb 14,496-foot-high Mount Whitney, backpack 40 miles into the Grand Canyon, or walk the Appalachian Trail.

One to whom television devoted considerable attention is Eula Weaver. At 85 years of age, Mrs. Weaver won two gold medals in the Senior Olympics at Irvine, California. It is her medical history that makes this performance all the more impressive. At the age of 67 she was treated for angina. At 75 she suffered a heart attack. By the age of 81 she had a variety of other medical problems. The following year she joined a group on a low-fat, low-cholesterol diet and started a planned exercise program. Her workout schedule called for running 1½ miles a day and pedaling the equivalent of 10 to 15 miles daily on a stationary bike as well as for two gym sessions a week. Her diet and exercise transformed Mrs. Eula Weaver into a Senior Olympics champion.

Feola Scharf is tall, brisk moving, gray-haired. She is a branch manager for one of New York City's major banks. About 30 years ago, when it was not too popular a sport, she started Alpine skiing. Several years ago she switched to cross-country skiing which is more demanding, more of a workout. Then she joined the Appalachian Mountain Club. Now, on those warm weekends when she is not bicycling or on the tennis courts, she hikes.

Recently Mrs. Scharf discovered jogging. She does her laps three or four times a week, either early in the morning before leaving for the bank or in the evening after work. Despite her already high level of cardiovascular and musculoskeletal fitness, she started running slowly, about 10 to 15 minutes a session with brief warm-up exercises before and after her workouts. Mrs. Scharf readily admits that "physical activity has become a way of life for me. I feel it has helped me maintain my equilibrium during stressful times."

Christiane Dickinson is a petite, charming Frenchwoman who has built a second life around jogging and marathon running. In her forties, she joined the Road Runners Club in New York City, attends their meetings, clinics, and Saturday morning exercise sessions, and competes in their runs. Mrs. Dickinson learned the importance of stretching and warm-up exercises early in her running. Running too fast without a warm-up in a short-distance event, she severely injured her Achilles tendon. But she did not quit the sport. Slowly, agonizingly, she worked her way back. Now she does not start working out without a full warm-up.

Mrs. Dickinson is one of the new breed of runners who take their training shoes with them when they travel. A sales executive for an international hotel chain, she regularly travels throughout the United States and Canada and Belgium. Somehow she finds the time to work out every day she is on the road.

Another woman who carries her running shoes wherever she goes is Helen Hatton, a free-lance home economist. I first met her on a Sunday morning when she ran past, looked back, and said, "Don't quit now." In her middle thirties, Miss Hatton is retained by major companies to travel the country and appear on television and radio programs. "When I first started asking hotel clerks where I could jog, they'd look at me as though I were from outer space. Now I find many of the hotels have a small track and gym, or little maps showing their guests how to get to the nearest park."

If you have young children, you have probably read Lynn Minton's movie recommendations in a major women's magazine. Mrs. Minton started running about six years ago when she realized she was "huffing on stairs and really out of condition." The convenience of jogging is important to her. When the pressures of meeting deadlines become too much, she gets into her running clothes and dashes across the street to a park. There she jogs about 1¾ miles, and then goes back to her typewriter. Mrs. Minton says: "One of the nice things about running is that it is completely uncomplicated: no arrangements, no reservations, no partners. Also I love it! I find it hard sometimes to get out, but when I do, I love doing it."

Running holds little appeal for Audrey McCaffrey, a sales promotion manager. She is a walker. On her job she walks from appointment to appointment at a pace that for many would be a jog. On weekends, she and her husband bike tour.

Molly Stark, a special projects editor for an outdoor magazine, has three major loves other than her family: hiking, white water canoeing, and canoe racing. All three demand high levels of physical and cardiovascular fitness.

Randee Rafkin-Rubin's work as a designer of annual reports and other sophisticated corporate printed materials is painstaking, often demanding twelve-hour days. To break free from the pressure of her work, she spends two evenings a week working on rings and uneven parallel bars in addition to jogging mornings and playing tennis on weekends. "I am amazed at seeing how quickly women in their sixties learn to work on the bars," Mrs. Rubin says. "When they begin, they often can't bend over far enough to touch their toes. But after several weeks, they loosen up and the next thing I see is they are working out with the rest of the class."

These women are busy, earning their livelihoods in a variety of demanding occupations. They are not athletes in the traditional meaning of the word, but they believe in the importance of consistent, vigorous exercise. Best of all, they enjoy their workouts.

Certainly age is no barrier and time can be made.

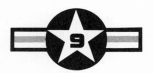

The Cardiovascular System

Only about the size of a fist, the heart is the sturdiest organ we have. An endurance muscle, it is superbly designed to pump our life-giving bloodstream through our many miles of arteries, capillaries, and veins.

The heart was shaped over the countless centuries when survival depended on the ability to run faster and farther than an enemy or attacking predator. Today, we still retain our fight-or-flight instinct— we feel it when we tense up during a crisis or argument—but that response has been dulled by civilization. Our lifestyle, often circumscribed by both desk and automobile, is frequently accused of being the heart's worst enemy. Slowed by inactivity and a body that often is overfed, the heart is exposed to the threat of the "lazy heart" syndrome. The myth of the athlete's enlarged heart caused by too much activity happily has been laid to rest. The condition just does not exist.

The more we work the healthy heart through training or physical activity, the better it functions, the more powerful it becomes. One immediately apparent result of conditioning is that the wind improves. You no longer gasp for breath after climbing a flight of stairs or running for a cab.

It has been found that as we exercise regularly, making the heart beat faster for extended periods of time, and as we gradually increase the demands placed on it, the heart muscle pumps a larger volume of blood with every beat. It becomes more efficient, thus able to slow its beat rate. It need no longer work as hard when we climb a hill or play a set of singles, just as an eight-cylinder car need not have gears shifted when climbing a hill while a four-cylinder may require a shift from high down to second. Your resting heartbeat rate may slow from a normal 72-74 beats per minute to 60, 50, and among some persons, to even fewer beats. This slowing down is called bradycardia, and when it is the result of exercise it is functional and no cause for concern. Careful monitoring has shown that over a period of 24 hours even moderate training can save your heart 10,000 to 20,000 heartbeats.

Your heart's increased efficiency helps it take activity in stride. Its beat rate may not climb as high as that of the deconditioned heart for the same amount of exertion. It also will return to its normal beat rate more quickly after exercise.

THE HEART, BLOOD VESSELS, AND LUNGS

The heart is made up of four chambers. The blood returning from the veins enters the right atrium, passes through the tricuspid valve into the right ventricle, and then is pumped through the pulmonary artery to the lungs where it is supplied with oxygen from the lungs.

From the lungs, the blood flows through the left atrium into the left ventricle and is pumped throughout the body via the aortic artery. The heart muscle receives blood through two small arteries located where the aorta leaves the heart.

The heart's rhythm is maintained and governed by its own built-in timing mechanism called the Sino-auricular (SA) node. During stress or excitement, the SA node raises the heartbeat, pumping a more rapid flow of oxygen-carrying blood through the body to meet the needs of the muscles and organs.

As it moves into the body, the aorta branches out into numerous arteries, and in turn into smaller arteries called arterioles, and finally into capillaries. It is in the body's network of minute capillaries—which are about 1/3000 of an inch in diameter—that the exchange is made with the body cells: the capillaries bring them nourishment and then collect cell wastes.

It is in the lungs and their one-billion-plus sacs called the alveoli that the body's oxygen/carbon dioxide exchange takes place. The oxygen molecules in the air that we inhale are passed through these alveoli into the capillaries, where they combine with the hemoglobin molecules in the red blood cells. The oxygen-carrying capacity of the red blood cells in women is about 19.0 milliliters of oxygen for each 100 milliliters of blood. This capacity can be affected by certain types of anemia and by menstruation.

If, while we are exercising or under stress, the heart cannot meet the demands made of it, the muscles do not receive the oxygen they need to maintain activity. We start breathing heavily, even over-breathing to maintain the oxygen flow. But we begin tiring. Eventually

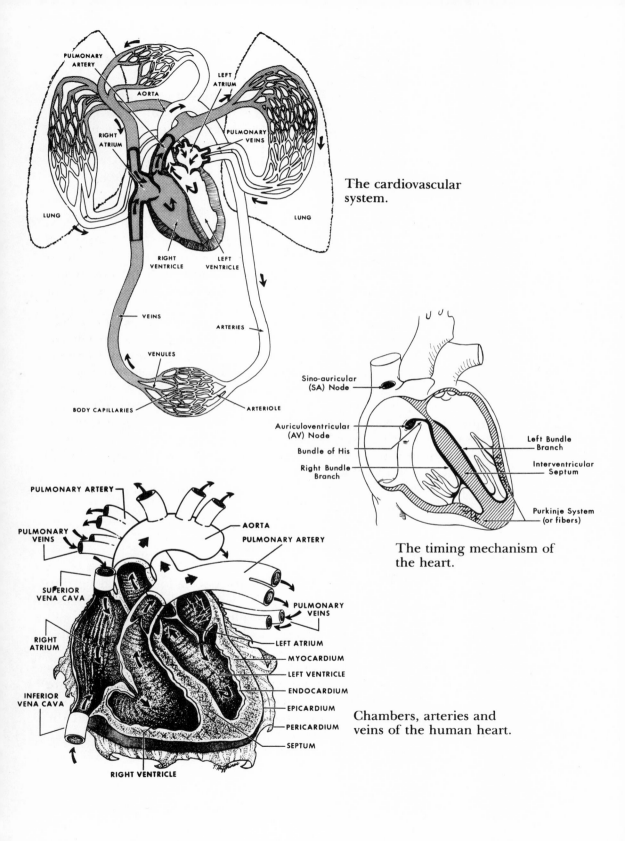

The cardiovascular system.

The timing mechanism of the heart.

Chambers, arteries and veins of the human heart.

we run out of breath and stop. Studies of muscles during strenuous exercise reveal a buildup of lactic acid, a significant by-product of muscle use which causes tiring, as well as a depletion of the muscles' stores of glycogen, a natural substance converted from carboyhydrates. This discovery led to the recent emphasis of carbohydrates in athletes' diet, about which more later.

THE RAMJET EFFECT

The ramjet engine is unique. The faster it goes, the faster it is able to go. There is an analogy here for you. The more your cardiovascular system is exercised, the more efficient it becomes, the harder it can work.

As you regularly work out at least three to four times a week over a period of months and even years, your cardiovascular system gains in efficiency and stamina. The heart's greater strength enables it to pump a higher volume of blood through the body with every stroke, and the result is a lowering of the resting heartbeat rate.

Training also tends to lower the resting blood pressure in some people. This, it is suggested, is due to the transient dilation of the body's vessels during exercise and, of lasting importance, an increase in the number and size of the arterioles and capillaries that supply blood to the skeletal muscles and the heart. This rise in vascularization may ameliorate a heart attack or reduce its severity, and may prove to be the difference between recovery and death.

JUDGING HEART RISK FACTORS

After extensive study, the American Heart Association evolved a group of risk factors that may be used to judge vulnerability to heart disease. These factors are by no means absolute. A low score does not guarantee invulnerability to heart attack. A high score does not imply that the worst is at hand.

They do help you to work out a balance sheet of your cardio-vascular assets and debits. Like entries in a balance sheet, some are subject to change and improvement.

The Cardio-Metrics Institute in New York has formulated the AHA risk factors into a self-scoring card you can use to arrive at an overall picture of your heart attack risk:

	(1)	(2)	(3)	(4)	(5)	(6)
Heredity	No heart disease in family (parents, sisters, brothers only)	One relative over 60 with heart attack	Two or more relatives over 60 with heart attack	One relative under 60 with heart attack	Two relatives under 60 with heart attack	Three or more relatives under 60 with heart attack
Blood Pressure	Low blood pressure	Normal blood pressure or don't know	High blood pressure only when upset	Mild high B.P. but no medication needed	High B.P. controlled by medication	High B.P. not completely controlled by medication
Diabetes	Low blood sugar	Normal blood sugar or don't know	Known high sugar controlled by diet	High sugar controlled by tablets	Diabetic on insulin— no complications	Diabetic complications (circulation, kidneys, eyes)
Smoking	Non-user or stopped permanently	Cigars or pipe only	Less than 5 cigarettes daily	6-20 cigarettes daily	21-39 cigarettes daily	Over 40 cigarettes daily
Weight	Five lbs. underweight to normal	Up to 5 lbs overweight	6-20 lbs overweight	21-35 lbs overweight	35-50 lbs overweight	51-65 lbs overweight

	(1)	(2)	(3)	(4)	(5)	(6)
Cholesterol	Below 180	181-205	206-230 or don't know	231-255	256-280	Over 281
Exercise	Very active physically in job & recreation	Moderately active in job & recreation	Sedentary job, very active in recreation	Sedentary job, moderately active recreation	Sedentary job, light recreation exercise	Complete lack of exercise
Emotional Stress	No real business or personal pressures	Rare business or personal pressure	Moderate business or personal pressures	Take pills or drink for stress on occasion	Constantly need pills or drink for stress	Intense problems, can't cope, see psychiatrist
Age	10-20	21-30	31-40	41-50	51-60	Over 60
Sex and Build	Female still menstruating	Male, thin build	Female after menopause	Male, build average	Male, fairly stocky	Male, very stocky

To determine your degree of risk, check off the box that applies to you on each line. Then total your number of points. Ten to 20 points indicate low risk; 21 to 40 moderate risk; 41 to 60 high risk.

When scoring yourself, forget the myth that only men are vulnerable to heart attack. It is true that compared with men, women are relatively well protected until late middle age, but not enough has been learned about the cardiovascular effects of business and other stresses to which women are now exposing themselves.

TESTING THE HEART

Your heart and your network of arteries, capillaries, and veins are a closed hydraulic system. A squeeze here, a block there, are reflected throughout the network.

The pulse is caused by the regular pumping of blood from the heart into the aorta, increasing and decreasing the pressure in that primary artery. As the blood races through the vessels, their walls expand and recoil giving the pulse the beat we can feel. The quickness or slowness of that pulse, its regularity or irregularity, steadiness or flutter, give sensitive physicians insight into their patients' emotional state as well as the health of their heart and vascular system.

Many of the popular songs we hear remind us that love makes the heart—and pulse—beat faster. That intercourse makes the heart beat faster has been confirmed by research. During orgasm the pulse rate nearly doubles, the stroke volume per beat is increased nearly 50 percent, and systolic pressure rises about 30 percent.

When we are excited or frightened, the blood seems to pound through the body. In turn, grief and depression may cause the pulse to beat slowly. Should heart or circulatory disease be present, the beat may be irregular or interrupted.

The pulse is also affected by tobacco and some foods. Smoking a pack of cigarettes can make the heart labor and the pulse race as though you are climbing innumerable flights of stairs. Foods you are allergic to also make the pulse speed up.

There are studies showing that a consistently higher pulse may be linked to a shorter life span. Statistical analysis of life insurance records reveals that policyholders with regular pulse rates of between 55 and 65 beats a minute have a 20 percent advantage in mortality over those with a pulse of about 70. Seventy is considered normal by many physicians. Infants have a normal beat of 110 to 140, and young children of 80 to 90. In old age, the pulse slows to about 60.

YOUR MAXIMUM PULSE RATE

There are physiological limits to how fast your heart can pump. At 20 years of age, your maximum heart rate is approximately 200 beats per minute. The rate decreases approximately one beat per minute per year past 20. At 30, the maximum rate is 190; at 35, 186; at 50, 175; and at 60, 168. Truly, age does slow us down.

The many years of research in human performance laboratories show that exercise carried on for extended periods of time at a heartbeat rate reaching 70 to 80 percent of the age-related maximum will have a strengthening effect. There are even indications that a badly deconditioned individual may benefit by exercising at 50 to 60 percent of her age-related maximum.

A number of tests have been used to measure cardiovascular fitness. One used for many years after World War II is the Harvard Step Test and its variations. This is a simple but strenuous procedure to check the heart's ability to cope with and then recover after strenuous physical activity. As simple as it is, its use should be approved by your physician and it should never be done while alone.

All that is needed is a low bench or wooden chair about 18 inches high. First you step up and down 24 times a minute for up to three minutes. After exercising, sit quietly and take your pulse for 30 seconds at intervals—from 1–1½ minutes, 2–2½ minutes, and 3–3½ minutes. There are several scoring criteria used to evaluate performance. One calls for the totaling of the three 30-second pulse counts. The result indicates your level of cardiovascular fitness. A total of more than 193 is poor; 176 to 187, fair; 158 to 170, average; 141 to 153, good; 126 to 135, excellent.

Many physicians followed the step test with an electrocardiogram (ECG). However, in the time it took to apply the ECG electrodes, the patient's heart rate slowed and the reading was basically of a heart at or near rest. While the standard resting ECG might bring to light major problems or indications of a silent heart attack, it does not answer the critical question of how the heart performs under stress.

The increased understanding of the exercise stress test and its capabilities finally took the procedure out of the performance laboratories into hospitals and private testing centers. Private testing centers may be found throughout the country. They not only test but also write exercise prescriptions to enhance cardiovascular fitness. These prescriptions may be rewritten periodically to keep pace with patients' improvement.

The exercise stress test currently is recognized as the most sensitive diagnostic or screening procedure available short of isotope studies and heart catheterization. In an article entitled "Why Take a Stress Test?" *Runner's World* magazine* carried an interview I did with Abner Delman, cardiologist and medical director; William Gualtiere, director; and Kerry J. Stewart, an exercise physiologist; all at Cardio-Metrics Institute. It answers many of the questions people have about exercise stress testing. What do doctors "see" when they wire you to an electrocardiograph machine while exercising? Can the tests help the mature, would-be fitness runner who is especially vulnerable to medical and physical problems? Are the tests really worth the time, effort, and money involved?

Doctors are sending patients for stress or exercise testing before they start training. Why not be satisfied with the resting ECG?

DELMAN: Let's take the analogy of a car that has been used primarily around the neighborhood or on an occasional run into the country. Under normal conditions it sounds well, performs well. But take it out at highway speeds for several hundreds of miles, and you may start hearing pings and noises you never suspected existed.

It's often the same with the heart. It may look good during an at-rest ECG, but when you make it really work for a period of time you may discover severe arrhythmias and other cardiac problems you did not know existed. Arrhythmias are variations from the normal rhythm of the heart. There is now evidence they can be forerunners of cardiac arrest.

If an individual comes of healthy stock, has no history of cardiac problems, shouldn't a good, routine examination be enough to give him a clean bill of health?

GUALTIERE: In general, I would say yes, particularly if he shows a good cardiac profile, normal blood pressure and blood lipids (fats) and so on. That reduces the risk of anything happening. But stress testing reduces that risk even further, particularly if the individual has been inactive over a period of years.

Is stress testing new?

GUALTIERE: About 50 years ago, it was called "performance testing." Over the years, considerable work was done in the laboratories dealing with the body processes and its response to physical stress. The data accumulated helped us place exercise programing on a rational or

---

*Reprinted with permission from *Runner's World* magazine.

objective basis. In fact, that work also has led to many of the better times we have seen in mile, cross-country and marathon.

When did testing leave the laboratory for general use?

DELMAN: Sometime in the mid-'50s with the use of exercise in the management of suspected or known cardiac patients. Since then it has gained in popularity, as do many new medical and health developments. But I think that is all to the good.

There has been some questioning of the entire procedure, though. For example, that the mere suggestion would-be runners take a test is enough to scare them off.

GUALTIERE: You can build a case for that point of view, I am sure. But you can also support the need for gaining as much cardiovascular data about individuals as possible before you let them start training. Our experience is that most people tend to overdo. They overstress and come down with all kinds of muscular and skeletal problems. Sometimes they come down with cardiac problems.

Let's face it, people sometimes die because they embark on a training program they shouldn't have undertaken. They thought they were all right. Most people who feel healthy usually don't see a physician—at least not until they have symptoms. The stress test, on the other hand, is capable of detecting early evidence of heart problems.

What does a typical stress test include?

GUALTIERE: We start by taking a comprehensive medical history of the individuals, with emphasis on cardiac incidents. We also check their report with their physician. Most of those we test are referred by physicians so that step isn't necessary. Then, if we believe we can safely test him, we start with a resting ECG. We're looking for anything new that might have developed since his last visit to a doctor.

DELMAN: Some people have silent heart attacks and don't know it. Assuming everything is in order after the initial work-up—blood pressure reading, ECG, etc.—we move on to the testing area.

During the stress test, we take a continuous ECG and monitor heart action at the same time on oscilloscopes. We also do a series of blood pressure readings and measure the body's oxygen-handling ability—all while the individual is exercising under increasing stress. We believe we're able to detect any available evidence of heart strain in this way. The test also gives us the data we need to develop a personalized exercise prescription for cardiac enhancement.

STEWART: We use electrically driven treadmills for our tests. This lets us control the belt's speed and also lets us tilt it at regular intervals. This makes the individual "climb a hill," causing his heart to work harder. His body also consumes more oxygen even though we keep the belt's speed constant. The more deconditioned the person is, the more quickly he'll peak out during the test. With those in better shape, the heart takes longer to reach the maximum beat rate we are targeting at during the stress period.

This way, we're able to quite accurately predict a person's maximum aerobic capacity. We don't have to test up to exhaustion, even though we have done so for some competitive runners. For the average person, we test up to at least 85 percent of maximum heartbeat rate. At that point, we slow the belt and start lowering it. We keep monitoring heart action and blood pressure and continue even when we get the individual off the belt and onto a chair. We want to detect any suspicious changes in the ECG that might appear only during the cool-down period. An abnormal response, for instance, might be an upsurge in blood pressure.

What happens after the test?

GUALTIERE: After we have had a chance to analyze the test, we bring the person back for a group session to explain our training philosophy. Then we review each person's exercise prescription individually so they can start training on a controlled basis.

What is your training philosophy?

GUALTIERE: Given an individual over 30 years of age who has been sedentary, our feeling is that of all the components associated with physical fitness, cardiovascular is most important. That is the cornerstone from which a fitness runner can go on to build muscle, improve flexibility, extensibility.

We also believe that interval training offers the best approach to beginning involvement with running. There are a number of reasons for this. Most important is that the older person's body will not permit exercise continuously at the necessary intensity, frequency, and duration to do good. Interval training eases people into running and builds them up to where they can phase into continuous training if they want.

STEWART: Even with younger people who might be able to skip the interval training phase, there is enough of a risk of coming down with muscular and skeletal problems to make it advisable to start with interval training. This lets runners gradually condition their bodies. They aren't wasting time; they are playing it safe.

GUALTIERE: Our sessions are divided into three stages—warm-up, stimulus, cool-down. It's in the stimulus stage that runners make their heart work, build up their fitness. We have them working at 75 to 85 percent of their maximum heartbeat rates. That's when the workout stimulates an improvement in their aerobic capacity.

A number of concepts have been advanced for conditioning the beginning runner. One is built on a point system. Another calls for a minimum run of six miles. The doctor who takes that approach says that any distance under six miles does little good.

DELMAN: It's not a matter of distance or of running against the clock. Our studies show that approximately 75-85 percent of individuals' age-related maximum heart rate must be attained if they are to benefit. Our objective is to help them enhance their cardiovascular fitness. This

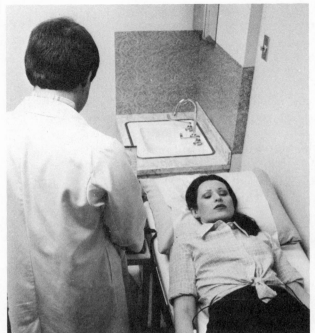

Taking an exercise stress test. When public relations executive Phyllis Melhado wished to start an intensive exercise program, she was referred to the Cardio-Metrics Institute for stress testing. After her medical history was taken, physiologist Garry Neupert did a resting cardiogram, and then took her blood pressure.

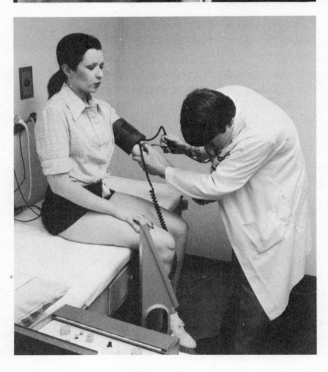

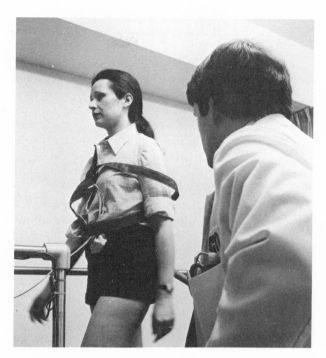

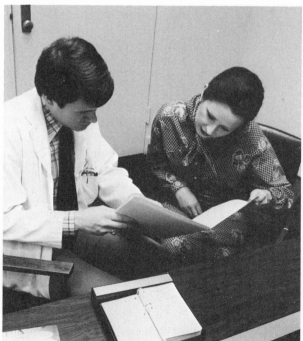

Following a stethoscopic examination by a cardiologist, she was exercised on an electric treadmill. The action of her heart as recorded on an oscilloscope and an ECG was monitored by the cardiologist during the test. After her tape was analyzed and she took part in a group seminar, her exercise prescription was discussed with her by Garry Neupert.
(Jack Galub photos)

calls for training 15-20 minutes at the target heart rate level, three to four times a week over a six- to nine-month period.

The training prescriptions we write for runners tell them when and how often they should count their pulse beats. That tells them if they are under- or over-stressing. We actually have them count their pulse for 10 seconds and then multiply by six. Not a particularly difficult task.

What about mature individuals who live in an area without testing facilities. What can they do?

DELMAN: They should seek the guidance of a physician. If that is impossible, they should become aware of the cardiac factors and should assess their own history against those factors. Then, if they have good cardiac profiles, they should start slowly. They must practice moderation from the very beginning. Should they at any time develop any unusual symptoms—chest pains, undue muscular soreness—they should stop.

GUALTIERE: For the first three weeks to a month they might limit themselves to walking. First, at a slow or moderate pace. Depending on age, brisk walking is all they may have to do to start rounding into shape. When they feel they have reached a peak in their walking, they might start jogging, using an interval approach. They are out to enhance their cardiovascular systems and to become fitness runners. They are not out there preparing for competition. If they want to go in that direction, that kind of training can come later.

STEWART: They should learn to keep their inner ear tuned to the body. If they are beginning to push too hard, their bodies and pulse rates will tell them. They should be willing to train consistently. We recommend stimulus periods of 15 to 20 minutes three times a week. Later on, if they want, they can increase the frequency of training periods. But they must remember they are no longer kids and must practice moderation.

HIGH BLOOD PRESSURE: NOT DRAMATIC, BUT DEADLY

Anne passed me easily, swinging around the turn at the far end of the reservoir. She looked back, shouted "Marathon coming up Saturday," and kept running.

Sixty yards later I caught up with her. She was leaning against the fence, pale, crying. She thought she was dying. Her leg muscles had quit working. She felt totally wrung out.

As I walked her home, she told me her physician had taken several readings over a year ago that showed her blood pressure was moderately high, and he had prescribed diuretics to be taken in the morning with orange juice. Suddenly she had stopped taking juice with the capsules, because the thought of all the calories bothered her. As a result, she later found out, her heart muscle started losing potassium; this is a common side effect of diuretics.

Potassium ions are important to a number of essential physiological processes. They help in the transmission of nerve impulses, the function of the cardiac, skeletal, and smooth muscle, and the maintenance of normal kidney functions.

Potassium lack is easily remedied. Increased use of foods high in potassium, such as orange juice, as well as the taking of potassium chloride tablets, will quickly restore potassium balance. (See table of potassium/sodium food values in this chapter.)

What Anne had found especially upsetting is that despite several years of intensive running she had become hypertensive. The disease had taken hold without symptoms. She had no headaches, no dizzy spells. She would not have known that she might have become an eventual stroke or heart attack candidate if she hadn't gone for a routine check-up.

The highly regarded Framingham Study, which has monitored 5,209 persons for more than 25 years, has confirmed that blood pressure is the dominant contributor to cardiovascular disease in the group studied. At any age, in either sex, risk has been shown to increase in proportion to the height of the blood pressure.

Over 23 million adult Americans are estimated to have high blood pressure. Of this group, 70 to 80 percent are considered borderline, with diastolic pressures of 90-104 mm Hg (millimeters of mercury). The diastolic—the lesser of the two numbers in a reading—measures the minimum pressure between heartbeats. The systolic—the higher of the numbers—measures the system's maximum pressure during contraction of the heart.

Treatment undertaken even with borderline patients,* some physicians believe, prevents the rise of pressure to dangerous levels and reduces the possibility of kidney damage or enlargement of the heart's left ventricle.

Many borderline patients are able to control their pressure by

---

*The National High Blood Pressure Education Program, U.S. Department of Health, Education, and Welfare, makes six general recommendations for detection, evaluation, and treatment of high blood pressure for adults. They include the recommendation that virtually all patients with a diastolic pressure of 105 or greater should be treated with antihypertensive drug therapy. For persons with diastolic pressures of 90-104, treatment should be individualized with consideration given to other risk factors.

stopping their use of birth control pills or by losing weight and restricting their salt intake. If not, diuretics may be prescribed. Then if pressure still is not brought under control, nerve-blocking drugs may be used in combination with the diuretics.

If adequate supplementary potassium is taken with diuretics, physical training usually can continue without difficulty, but be extra careful in hot, humid weather to protect against heatstroke. The nerve-blocking drugs, however, slow the heart itself, thus relieving pressure on the vascular system. Then exercise is affected. Running while taking the drugs has been described as trying to drive a car in high gear with the brakes on.

No matter which drugs your physician prescribes, the chances are you will be told to exercise to maintain body tone. If you cannot run, then swim or walk. You should keep your body active and fit.

ALTERNATIVE APPROACHES TO HYPERTENSION

That mind and personality may contribute to high systolic readings has not been overlooked by psychiatrists. Some clinicians believe that in some patients essential hypertension (hypertension without any direct traceable organic cause) may be the result of sustained emotional tension caused by personality problems. They hold that those persons may be passive, less than normally assertive people who bottle up their anger. They are endlessly trying to please others while suppressing feelings of anger and aggression. They may also be described as uncomfortable if their affairs are not in meticulous order.

Joan, a family service social worker, says she decided to cope with her high blood pressure in her own way. She bought a variety of books dealing with biofeedback, meditation, and mind control and eventually found an approach she was comfortable with. She also purchased a blood pressure kit and had her physician instruct her in its use.

She kept a log of her readings whenever she did something significant during the day. She found that some staff meetings sent her readings climbing, but that she could control them by closing her office door and meditating for fifteen minutes or so. She discovered her pressure rose when she spoke on the telephone with certain friends. She reduced the frequency and length of those calls. She eliminated sodium from her diet and lost weight. Today, she says, her physician does not believe the low readings he takes of her pressure and wants her to continue medication. She has refused and so far has maintained a completely normal blood pressure.

Biofeedback and transcendental meditation have been found to reduce blood pressure. Dr. Herbert Benson's book, *The Relaxation Response*, presents another meditation-like approach that offers the possibility of lower readings. His method calls for the person to sit passively in a quiet room with eyes closed and, while breathing through the nose, to say the word "one" silently while inhaling and then again when exhaling. He recommends two 10- to 20-minute sessions a day.

Dr. Donald L. Wilson's system, which he describes in his book *Total Mind Power,* is designed to let you use the 90 percent of the mind that is virtually untapped to help lower blood pressure and cope with other problems. His is a three-step approach calling for first, a focusing of awareness, then a directing of the mind, and finally a sequencing of the mind's direction to arrive at the proper repetition of the first two steps.

A caution: If you are on medication and wish to explore a mind control system, discuss your objectives with your physician. It probably will be suggested that you first master the system you choose and that you taper off your medication gradually. Periodic blood pressure readings should be taken to make certain your pressure remains controlled.

HIGH-POTASSIUM—LOW-SODIUM FOODS

	Portion	Potassium (mg.)	Sodium (mg.)
Apple juice	6 oz	187	2
Coca-Cola	6 oz	88	2
Coffee (brewed)	1 cup	149	3
Orange juice			
Fresh	8 oz	496	3
Canned	8 oz	500	3
Prune juice	6 oz	423	4
Apples	1 medium	165	1
Apricots			
Fresh	2–3	281	1
Canned (in syrup)	3 halves	234	1
Dried	17 halves	979	26
Bananas	1 6-in	370	1
Blueberries	1 cup	81	1
Cantaloupe	¼ melon	251	12
Cherries			
Fresh	½ cup	191	2
Canned (in syrup)	½ cup	124	1
Dates			
Fresh	10 medium	648	1
Dried (pitted)	1 cup	1150	2
Fruit cocktail	½ cup	161	5
Grapefruit	½ medium	135	1

HIGH-POTASSIUM—LOW-SODIUM FOODS

	Portion	Potassium (mg.)	Sodium (mg.)
Grapes	22 grapes	158	3
Oranges	1 small	200	1
Peaches			
Fresh	1 medium	202	1
Canned	2 halves	130	2
Pears			
Fresh	½ pear	130	2
Canned	2 halves	84	1
Pineapple			
Fresh	¾ cup	146	1
Canned	1 slice	96	1
Plums			
Fresh	2 medium	299	2
Canned	3 medium	142	1
Prunes			
Dried	10 large	694	8
Strawberries	10 large	164	1
Watermelon	½ cup	100	1
Artichoke			
Base and soft end of leaves	1 large bud	301	30
Asparagus			
Fresh	⅔ cup	183	1
Canned	6 spears	191	271
Beans, baked	⅝ cup	704	2
Beans, green			
Fresh	1 cup	189	5
Canned	1 cup	109	295
Beans, lima			
Fresh	⅝ cup	422	1
Canned	½ cup	255	271
Frozen	⅝ cup	394	129
Beets			
Fresh	½ cup	172	36
Canned	½ cup	138	196
Broccoli	⅔ cup	267	10
Brussels sprouts	6–7 medium	273	10
Cabbage			
Raw, shredded	1 cup	233	20
Cooked	⅗ cup	163	14
Carrots			
Raw	1 large	341	47
Cooked	⅔ cup	222	33
Canned	⅔ cup	120	236
Cauliflower	⅞ cup	206	9
Celery	1 outer or 3 inner stalks	170	63

HIGH-POTASSIUM—LOW-SODIUM FOODS

	Portion	Potassium (mg.)	Sodium (mg.)
Corn			
Fresh	1 medium ear	196	trace
Canned	½ cup	81	196
Cucumber, pared	½ medium	80	3
Lettuce, iceberg	3½ oz	264	9
Mushrooms (uncooked)	10 small, 4 large	414	15
Onions (uncooked)	1 medium	157	10
Peas			
Fresh	⅔ cup	196	1
Canned	¾ cup	96	236
Frozen	3½ oz	135	115
Potatoes			
Boiled (in skin)	1 medium	407	3
French fried	10 pieces	427	3
Radishes	10 small	322	18
Sauerkraut	⅔ cup	140	747
Tomatoes			
Raw	1 medium	366	4
Canned	½ cup	217	130
Paste	3½ oz	888	38
Bacon	1 strip	16	71
Beef			
Corned beef (canned)	3 slices	51	803
Hamburger	¼ pound	382	41
Pot roast (rump)	½ pound	309	43
Sirloin steak	½ pound	545	57
Frankfurter (all beef)	⅛ lb	110	550
Chicken (broiled)	3½ oz	320	78
Duck	3½ oz	285	82
Ham			
Fresh	¼ lb	260	37
Cured, butt	¼ lb	239	518
Cured, shank	¼ lb	155	336
Lamb			
Shoulder chop (1)	½ lb	422	72
Rib chop (2)	½ lb	398	68
Leg roast	¼ lb	246	41
Liver			
Beef	3½ oz	325	86
Calf	3½ oz	436	131
Pork			
Loin chop	6 oz	500	52
Spareribs (3 or 4)	3½ oz	360	51
Sausage (link or bulk)	3½ oz	140	740
Turkey	3½ oz	320	40

HIGH-POTASSIUM—LOW-SODIUM FOODS

	Portion	Potassium (mg.)	Sodium (mg.)
Veal			
Cutlet	6 oz	448	46
Loin chop (1)	½ lb	384	54
Rump roast	¼ lb	244	36
Clams	4 large		
	or 9 small	235	36
Cod	3½ oz	382	70
Flounder or sole	3½ oz	366	56
Lobster (1) boiled, with 2 tbsp. butter	¾ lb	180	210
Oysters (5 to 8)			
Fresh	3½ oz	121	73
Frozen	3½ oz	210	380
Salmon (pink, canned)	3½ oz	361	387
Sardines (canned in oil)	3½ oz	560	510
Shrimp	3½ oz	220	140
Tuna			
Canned, in oil	3½ oz	301	800
Canned, in water	3½ oz	279	41
Candy			
Chocolate creams	1 candy	15	15
Milk chocolate	1 oz	105	30
Ice cream			
Chocolate	½ pint	*	75
Vanilla	½ pint	210	82
Nuts			
Cashews (roasted)	6–8	84	2
Peanuts (roasted)			
Salted	1 tbsp	105	69
Unsalted	1 tbsp	111	trace
Olives			
Green	2 medium	7	312
Ripe	2 large	5	150
Potato chips	5 chips	88	34
Pretzels (3 ring)	1 average	7	87
Butter			
(salted)	1 pat	2	99
(unsalted)	1 pat	2	1
Cheese			
American, cheddar	1 oz	23	197
American, processed	1 oz	22	318
Cottage, creamed	3½ oz	85	229
Cream (heavy)	1 tbsp	10	35

*Not available

HIGH-POTASSIUM—LOW-SODIUM FOODS

	Portion	Potassium (mg.)	Sodium (mg.)
Egg	1 large	70	66
Milk (whole)	8 oz	352	122
Oleomargarine (salted)	1 pat	2	99
Bread			
Rye	1 slice	33	128
White (enriched)	1 slice	20	117
Whole wheat	1 slice	63	121
Corn flakes	1 cup	40	165
Macaroni (enriched, cooked)	1 cup	85	1
Noodles (enriched, cooked)	1 cup	70	3
Oatmeal (cooked)	1 cup	130	1
Rice (white, dry)	¼ cup	45	3
Spaghetti (enriched, cooked)	1 cup	92	2
Waffles (enriched)	1 waffle	109	356
Wheat germ	3 tbsp	232	1

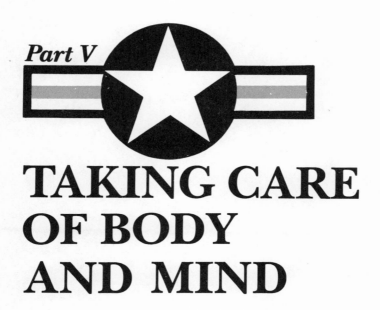

Part V

TAKING CARE
OF BODY
AND MIND

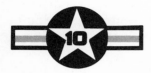

Travel and Exercise

Increased business travel, package tours, and low-tourist fares offer the chance to hike, run, swim, and bicycle far from home. Therefore, travelers today pack their sports equipment as a matter of course. But exercise at altitudes or temperatures you are not accustomed to may cause serious problems.

COPING WITH HEAT

Heat in some ways is more of a hazard than cold. Dr. James F. Knochel, professor of internal medicine at the University of Texas Southwestern Medical School at Dallas and an expert on heat injuries, points out that death from heatstroke is more common than statistics show. The deaths are often ascribed to something other than heatstroke because they are preventable and their "occurrence is embarrassing."

The two types of heatstroke he discusses are called "exertional" and "classic." Exertional heatstroke is caused by heat generated during muscle activity, that is, exercise or work; the heat accumulates faster than the body can dissipate it. Classic heatstroke can occur with or without exertion and usually is caused by the inability of the circulatory system to respond to heat stress; not enough perspiration is produced to cool the body.

The heart is the key to your ability to cope with heat. It must increase its output so it can pump the hot blood to the skin surface, where the heat is dissipated by sweating. If the heart does not respond properly or if the blood volume is low as in dehydration, then the sweat mechanism will fail and the body temperature will climb.

Humidity is a major contributor to heatstroke. If the air is saturated, sweat will not evaporate. Perspiration that rolls off or drips does not cool the body. If your body is completely covered in hot weather or if you are wearing a weight-loss suit, you can easily get into

155

trouble. The same is true for a woman who is taking diuretics that decrease body fluids. It is dangerous for her to exercise strenuously in the heat because her blood volume is inadequate.

Prevention should be your goal. Even if you are fully acclimated, it is safer to work in the early morning or late afternoon when sun and heat are less intensive. Dress lightly and comfortably, and drink plenty of water before, during, and after exercising.*

Once you start perspiring, your total body fluid content begins to deplete. As fluid loss increases, mental alertness and physical response decrease. Researchers have found that such depletion can lead to death even in cool climates:

Percent of Loss	Effect
2½	Dehydration begins
5	Nausea
6–10	Giddiness, headaches, limbs itch
15	Death imminent in 90° weather
25	Death even in cool climates

Dr. Knochel also points out that taking salt tablets before exercise is highly dangerous. Dehydration can cause the salt concentration in the blood to go extremely high and "the excess salt draws water out of the brain, turning it into a prune." Salt and other electrolytes lost from the body during heat can be restored during meals as part of a balanced diet.

A person suffering from just heat exhaustion will be sweating and may still be conscious. Usually they feel weak and just need water and rest. Someone with heatstroke, however, is in a coma and unresponsive to external stimulation. Sweating usually stops, so the skin is dry, flushed, and extremely hot to touch. The body temperature usually climbs above 106°. If body temperature reaches 108°, the possibility of permanent brain damage looms. Immediate first aid is imperative, even before the ambulance arrives. Get the victim out of the sun, remove clothes, douse him or her with water. Use a piece of clothing or whatever is available to fan the person and start the sweat evaporating to cool the skin.

---

*The Marine Corps has adopted the Israeli "overdrink" system to avoid heat problems. Marines must drink water at least every hour, and every 30 minutes when active in hot weather. Air Force survival training recommends drinking water as you need it. When running, playing tennis, or engaging in other active sports, do not let yourself dehydrate.

COPING WITH COLD

Body warmth is generated in the torso as a product of metabolic action and is carried by the bloodstream to the arms, legs, and head. When heat loss begins to build up at these points, the blood vessels constrict, cutting down the flow of blood so the torso may be protected. Your feet and fingers become uncomfortably cold, your nose turns blue, your ears start hurting. Shivering sets in, an instinctive reaction that steps up the heart's pumping action and the flow of blood. Goose bumps dot your body.

For backpacking and camping, as well as cross-country and Alpine skiing, the military triad approach to preparing troops for cold weather should be followed:

- An outer shell, tightly woven and water-repellent to protect inner, layered insulation from wind and rain.
- Insulation or layers to reduce heat loss. By adjusting the amount of layers worn you can regulate heat, retaining it against the body or allowing it to escape, to adjust to temperature changes. Layering is the most effective form of insulation commonly used. Several layers of medium-weight, loosely fitting clothing are more effective than one heavy garment as thick or thicker than the combined layers.
- Ventilation to keep body temperature level and let perspiration evaporate. Trapped perspiration fills your clothing with moisture, reducing its ability to keep you warm. The simplest way to cool an overheated part of the body is to open cuffs or collars, or to take off a layer of clothing.

If you are to be exposed to the bone-chilling weather of mountain altitudes or snow-belt regions for any extended period, your first layer of clothing should be cotton underwear worn under long johns. Quilted Dacron is worn in deep cold country, and double-layered cotton underwear in more temperate areas. Wool-blend shirts and pants are preferable, and over them a water-repellent hunting jacket or parka with a removable insulating layer. Most ski clothing is designed for this specialized sport and may not provide the protection needed for other activities.

The military advocates wearing one pair of padded wool-blend socks, instead of the two tighter fitting pairs suggested by some. The single pair does not fill up the warm air pockets inside your boots.

Mittens are suggested as warmer than conventional fingered gloves. There also are battery-warmed mittens on the market you might consider using.

For face protection against wind there are ski masks which are excellent when used with a Scottish balaclava or knitted wool hat.

The problem of cold weather jogging is somewhat different from such winter sports as skiing. Use common sense. If the weather is too cold for comfortable breathing, find an indoor track or gym to run in. You might also jog at home. Most women are comfortable wearing a lined sweat suit or lined warm-up suit with long johns underneath, along with wool mittens and knit hat. A little experience will tell you when long johns are needed.

Do not overdress. The great enemy of cold weather warmth is perspiration, as well as soiled outer clothes. Wet and soil are cold conductors. I find it best to dress lightly and let the heat generated by my body during running or cross-country skiing keep me warm.

Traditionally the insulation of choice for parkas, jackets, and sleeping bags is down. When dry, down is excellent: it's light, warm, and easily packed. When wet, though, it clumps, loses the protection it offers, and becomes a nuisance to dry. As a result, some outfitters sell rain and jackets to wear over down garments.

The use of down recently was set back by the tripling of its price and the difficulty of finding inexpensive garments that meet Federal standards. This led to the introduction of excellent man-made insulation for use in outerwear, including Celanese Fortrel PolarGuard and DuPont "Dacron" Hollofill.

The newest insulating material to come on the market is 3M Thinsulate Thermal Insulation. The manufacturer believes that on the surface of every insulation fiber there is a thin coating or layer of air which is held there by friction. The smaller the diameter or size of the fibers, and the more fibers in a given space, the higher the thermal resistance of the material. It is these air layers that provide the warmth needed in cold weather. 3M tests have shown that their insulation is almost twice as warm as equal amounts of down.

WIND CHILL FACTOR: NOT JUST TV TALK

Wind chill factor or "equivalent chill temperature" means more than a few seconds of talk on TV weather reports. Cold weather combined with even a moderate wind can cause flesh to freeze rapidly. As the above chart indicates, a temperature of 20°F. will have the same effect

Cooling Power of Wind Expressed as "Equivalent Chill Temperature"

Wind Speed (Knots)	(MPH)	Temperature (F) — Equivalent Chill Temperature																				
		40	35	30	25	20	15	10	5	0	−5	−10	−15	−20	−25	−30	−35	−40	−45	−50	−55	−60
Calm	Calm	40	35	30	25	20	15	10	5	0	−5	−10	−15	−20	−25	−30	−35	−40	−45	−50	−55	−60
3-6	5	35	30	25	20	15	10	5	0	−5	−10	−15	−20	−25	−30	−35	−40	−45	−50	−55	−65	−70
7-10	10	30	20	15	10	5	0	−10	−15	−20	−25	−35	−40	−45	−50	−60	−65	−70	−75	−80	−90	−95
11-15	15	25	15	10	0	−5	−10	−20	−25	−30	−40	−45	−50	−60	−65	−70	−80	−85	−90	−100	−105	−110
16-19	20	20	10	5	0	−10	−15	−25	−30	−35	−45	−50	−60	−65	−75	−80	−85	−95	−100	−110	−115	−120
20-23	25	15	10	0	−5	−15	−20	−30	−35	−45	−50	−60	−65	−75	−80	−90	−95	−105	−110	−120	−125	−135
24-28	30	10	5	0	−10	−20	−25	−30	−40	−50	−55	−65	−70	−80	−85	−95	−100	−110	−115	−125	−130	−140
29-32	35	10	5	−5	−10	−20	−30	−35	−40	−50	−60	−65	−75	−80	−90	−100	−105	−115	−120	−130	−135	−145
33-36	40	10	0	−5	−15	−20	−30	−35	−45	−55	−60	−70	−75	−85	−95	−100	−110	−115	−125	−130	−140	−150

Winds Above 40 Have Little Additional Effect.

Little Danger

Increasing Danger
(Flesh may freeze within 1 minute)

Great Danger
(Flesh may freeze within 30 seconds)

Danger of Freezing Exposed Flesh for Properly Clothed Persons

Source: Air Force Survival Manual

on your body as −10° in a 16 mph wind. When the temperature or equivalent chill temperature drops to −25° or less the flesh may freeze within one minute.

You should use the chart to help you decide how to dress for the outdoors and—more important—to help you decide when not to take part in outdoor activities unless you are prepared for the cold and wind.

FREEZING OR FROSTBITE

Frostbite or the freezing of flesh is caused by exposure to below-freezing temperatures, especially when winds are strong. At first there is an uncomfortable sensation of coldness followed by numbness. There may be a tingling, stinging, or aching, even a cramp-like pain. The skin first turns red. Later it becomes pale gray or waxy white.

Should you feel these sensations in your feet, react immediately. If you are near rocks, start kicking your feet against them. If you have a dry pair of socks, take off your boots or shoes immediately, peel off your wet socks and massage your feet with the dry pair before putting them on. If your hands show signs of extreme chill, pound them together to get the blood circulating and then shove them deep into a pocket or even under your jacket to keep them warm.

Do not wait until you are past the uncomfortable stage, until you have frostbite. Then you may have to be carried to shelter on a litter.

COPING WITH ALTITUDE

The effects of altitude vary, but they can be insidious. Happy-go-lucky tourists will deplane in Mexico or Switzerland, breathe deeply, feel euphoric, and then discover it almost impossible to ski or work out. Some travelers report they are ill, sluggish, sleepy, even suffer nosebleeds at altitudes. Others have little initial discomfort, only to discover their third day is marked by extreme fatigue.

Once an adjustment is made, the effects can be impressive. Captain Sherry Smith says that now when she is away from the Academy and plays tennis at sea level, she can go an extra set or two without difficulty. Her heightened stamina lasts some three weeks. When she returns to the Academy, it takes a while before she can function physically as well as before she left.

Few researchers have the opportunity to study the female and male athlete as closely as Major Philip R. Elliott, director of the Human Performance Laboratory at the Academy. Dr. Elliott received his doctorate in physical education at the University of New Mexico for his dissertation, *A Comparison of Males and Females During Acute Exposure to Hypobaria* (diminished oxygen supply). He and Dr. Hemming A. Atterbom tested 17 male and 20 female college students in a pressure chamber. Initial testing on a bicycle ergometer was at an altitude of 1,576 meters, to which all were acclimated. Afterward, the group was tested in a chamber at simulated altitudes of 2,743 meters and 3,962 meters.

These studies indicated that the major difference between women and men at altitude lies in the disparity of ventilation, the quantity of air women and men can breathe in and out. Women were unable to increase their ventilation during exercise at altitude, while men could. It is possible that women are able to function easily at lower altitudes because they may normally have good local blood perfusion in their active muscles without having to increase their heart rates.

You may find that altitude only briefly reduces your endurance, or it may cause high altitude sickness. Should you make an adjustment, you probably will find that the stamina built up at height gives you an edge when you return home.

That increased ability is due not so much to any buildup of hemoglobin caused by living in higher altitudes for a long time, Major Elliott explains, as it is to the training stress itself. The very act of training at altitude makes the heart work harder, adds stress. Overall that results in a more effective and more intensive conditioning program.

But time is needed to acclimate. Despite her superb conditioning, Olympic ice skating champion Anne Henning found it difficult to adjust to high altitude running. She eased into it, built up gradually.

The Denver YMCA sponsors the Mt. Evans run, a grueling 14.2 miles which begin at an elevation of 10,600 feet and ends at the 14,200-feet-high summit. Trophies are awarded to men who finish in under 2 hours and 40 minutes, and to women who do the run in under 3 hours. Despite the climb and the altitude, the starting field has grown from 17 in 1971 to several hundred. Nearly all runners last the distance and about one-half qualify for trophies.

Robb Hermanson of the Y athletic staff recommends that even seasoned runners take four months to prepare for Mt. Evans and similar marathons. "I'd do level work here in Denver and then portions of the mountain. Almost inevitably, you will find you will have to rebuild your cardiovascular endurance."

HIGH ALTITUDE SICKNESS

Most visitors to moderate and higher altitudes find that after a brief period of discomfort, they are able to function well if they take time to acclimate to the thinner air. However, some suffer some form of high altitude sickness.

Mountain Sickness: Before becoming ill, the new arrival at moderately high elevations (3,000 to 4,000 meters) usually feels well for the first few hours. A feeling of exhilaration is not unusual. There may be an initial awareness of breathlessness upon exertion and a need for frequent pauses to rest. Breathing irregularities can occur, particularly during sleep. The true onset of symptoms begins four to twelve hours after arrival at the higher altitude, with feelings of sickness, sluggishness, headache. Headache is the most distressing symptom and may be quite severe. Even when headache is not present, there is almost always some loss of appetite and decrease in tolerance for food. Vomiting may occur, contributing toward dehydration. Symptoms usually develop and increase to a peak intensity by the second day and they gradually subside over the next several days so that the total course may extend five to seven days.

Treatment consists of relieving the headache with aspirin or an equivalent. The patient should wear sunglasses since bright sunlight seems to aggravate the headache. The patient should be reassured, encouraged to take light foods and fluids. The symptoms may be alleviated by moving the patient to lower altitudes.

High Altitude Pulmonary Edema (HAPE): This may be considered a form of acute mountain sickness. It is characterized by high mortality. The incidence of HAPE, fortunately, is much less frequent than mountain sickness. Cases usually occur within 24 to 60 hours after arrival at altitude. Contributing factors include history of prior HAPE, a rapid or abrupt transition to high altitude, strenuous physical activity, exposure to cold, and anxiety.

HAPE symptoms include a progressive dry cough which develops frothy white or pink sputum. Cyanosis, the turning blue of the face, hands, and feet, will occur and become more intense. Patients with acute mountain sickness should be watched closely for increasing ill feeling, labored breathing, repeated clearing of the throat, development of the dry cough, and an increase in difficult or labored breathing at night. In rapidly progressive cases the onset of respiratory difficulty may be quite sudden, associated with a choking feeling and rapid deterioration in the ability to breathe.

Treatment includes rest, warmth, and the administration of oxygen; the patient should be immediately evacuated to lower altitudes if possible. If untreated, HAPE may become irreversible.

Dr. Borisse B. Paulin, an internist and cardiologist at the Lenox Hill Hospital in New York City, preaches common sense to help avoid altitude sickness. "Don't start running as soon as you get off the plane unless you are there to compete. Spend a few days becoming acclimated. Before you leave home, talk with your personal physician about the possible use of medication you may need at altitude."

The use of medication to help prevent mountain sickness is still being questioned by some physicians. It is wiser to spend time acclimating yourself to altitude before taking part in strenuous activity. Should you show any of the symptoms described, check with a physician and be prepared to move to a lower altitude if necessary.

COPING WITH WATER EMERGENCIES

Many warm-water swimming and boating tragedies might have been avoided if the victims had known how to "drownproof" themselves.

Drownproofing is taught by the American Red Cross, in Y's, and by professional swimming instructors. It is easily learned by swimmers, and nonswimmers learn to swim more quickly after learning the technique. Drownproofing makes use of the body's natural buoyancy and tendency to hang in a semi-vertical position in water, head just breaking the surface.

It is best learned at poolside, where the correct position—head bent forward, arms down but slightly extended from the body to the side, legs together—can easily be practiced. With the help of a friend, kneel on the bottom of the pool at the shallow end. Tilt the head back to bring nose and mouth above the surface to inhale fresh air, then tilt forward to exhale. Finally, go into deeper water and practice the standing-up position. You will find that your natural buoyancy will bring you up to the surface. Bring your face above the surface only when you really need a breath, then sink back into the drownproof position. Practice until you can stay afloat an hour.

Survival is extremely difficult in cold water. Anything below 70° F. is classified as "cold" by the Coast Guard; this temperature causes heat loss from the body. When the body's core temperature drops below its normal 98.6° F., surface tissues cool quickly, and the victim may experience labored breathing and stiffness of limbs and hands. At 95° there will be violent shivering; at 95° to 90° mental faculties slow; at 90° to 86° muscular rigidity and loss of consciousness set in. Below 86° there is possible heart failure and below 80° respiration becomes almost undetectable and death is imminent.

Research by the University of Victoria in Canada indicates that survival in 50° F. water is increased by extra body fat and decreased by small body size. Although women generally possess slightly more fat than men, they cool about 15 percent faster on the average because of their smaller body size. Children, because of their smaller body size, cool much faster than adults.

The Coast Guard has found that in many so-called drownings the cause of death actually was a progressive drop in the body's core temperature or hypothermia.

When boating on cold water, the Coast Guard recommends wearing a PFD (Personal Flotation Device). If thrown overboard, try to keep your lungs filled with air to maintain buoyancy; use a minimum of movement to prevent the escape of trapped air in your clothing; take advantage of floating paddles or debris for buoyancy, and maintain the HELP (Heat Escape Lessening Position) posture.

HELP is designed to extend survival time. You merely pull up your knees toward your chest while your arms are crossed over your chest. If several persons are in the water they should cling together in a huddle formation. Both positions are meant to help slow the loss of body heat and improve the chances of survival until help arrives.

Experience shows that swimming for shore is almost an impossibility if you are any distance away. Some good swimmers have been able to swim eight-tenths of a mile in 50° F. water before being overcome by hypothermia. Others have not been able to swim 100 yards. Therefore, do not swim unless there is absolutely no chance of rescue and you are absolutely certain you can make it. If you decide to swim, use a PFD or other flotation aid.

Kapok life jackets and loose-fitting foam vest-type life jackets provide no significant protection. Protection is increased by close-fitting vests and garment-type flotation jackets using buoyant, insulative foam between inner and outer layers of fabric. Even more protection is provided by a survival suit which uses foam in the legs and by the University of Victoria-developed UVic Thermofloat, a survival suit that allows trapping of water within insulative foam over the major heat loss areas of the body.

Aches, Pains, Bruises, and Other Matters

As long as major muscle groups are used to exercise the body, cardiovascular fitness is enhanced. The body little knows or cares whether you are swimming, running, playing tennis or handball, as long as your workouts are sufficiently intensive and continue long enough to make your heart work adequately.

For many women, cardiovascular stamina comes easily. Their heart is called on to power a smaller body, smaller muscles, and lighter bones, so when asked to perform, it often can.

That may be why you often see women looking more at ease than men when working out. That also may be why many women make the six-mile runs really fun. Other than the few in the lead who have worked on speed training and are there to beat the pack, many look at the races as social occasions, chatting with each other as their legs eat up the miles.

Some people's quick conditioning means their stamina outpaces their bodies' conditioning and this may cause problems. They tend to do too much too soon and too often collect more than their share of injuries.

The Air Force Academy found that women's injuries tend to cluster in the lower parts of the body—legs, ankles, feet, knees. If they play gymnastics or tennis they may expose themselves to knee or elbow damage. A number of elements contribute to this tendency. The lightness of women's bones makes them susceptible to fractures and joint injuries as well as strains and sprains. And if an ankle is sprained during premenstruum, the normal increase in tissue fluid may slow healing dramatically.

Adding to the inherent physiological aspects of injury are the shoes women normally wear. Higher heels and lack of foot support

165

limit body movement. Seldom is a woman seen running on the street unless she is dressed for jogging. Her shoes' higher heels tend to shorten her Achilles tendons' extensibility. If she starts running too fast too soon, she may pull or even snap a tendon. The regular use of high-heeled shoes also causes tight calves which can lead to shin splints, common among beginning runners.

Women's wider pelvises bring pressure on knees and ankles, opening them to foot and knee injuries, particularly in sports that demand explosive power. Gymnastics, competitive swimming and bicycling, and long-distance running in improperly fitted or designed shoes can bring on knee problems, especially if the woman overstresses or overuses her body without preliminary weight training and warm-up exercises. Some physicians also believe women may be more prone than men to tennis elbow because their forearms just are not as strong as they might be.

While a flexible body does well on the balance beam and in yoga and ballet, that suppleness also opens it to injury. If you can place the palms of both hands on the floor while keeping arms and legs straight, if you can turn your feet out while standing so they make an almost straight line, and if you can sit in the full lotus position, you are highly flexible.

Strength exercises will help you protect your muscles, ligaments, and joints. If you are not particularly supple, you should emphasize your stretching exercises to make your body more limber.

Warm-up exercises should be considered a must before any workout to prepare your body and cardiovascular system for the work they will be doing. It usually is the novice or overconfident athlete who decides warm-ups and cool-downs are wastes of time. As a result, they often are forced to endure the pain of cramps or, worse, of muscle or tendon tears.

The beginner who eases into her sports, gradually building up body tone and strengthening the muscle groups used in her activities, who does her flexibility and warm-up exercises faithfully, will reduce her danger of injury. But there is a tendency to overdo, and strains and sprains do happen.

For most such run-of-the-mill injuries, cryotherapy, that is, the use of ice, may be a woman's best friend, suggests Holly Wilson of the University of Iowa athletic department.

Miss Wilson was the first woman to complete the Athletic Training Specialization at Indiana State University and one of the first women to be certified by the National Athletic Trainers Association.

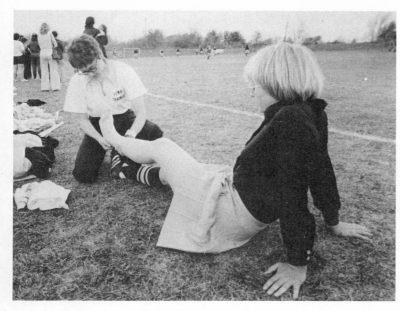

Holly Wilson at work on
the University of Iowa
playing field.
(Drake Hokanson photo)

She served as trainer for the 1970 World Games Trials in Gymnastics
and the 1972 Olympic Trials in Gymnastics. At the University of Iowa
she is a trainer working with both women's and men's teams.

She points out that muscle soreness from exercise experienced
by newcomers to intensive activity is the result of a buildup of metabolic
by-products in the muscles. Usually this soreness appears several hours
after the first workouts. The best way to alleviate this type of soreness is
to maintain a regular exercise program, letting your body adapt to
activity.

Pain that occurs during training often indicates damage to
tissue—a "pulled muscle" or strain. The severity of the injury depends
on the number of muscle fibers damaged during exercise. With the
tearing of tissue, there is bleeding into the area and swelling.

Ice should be applied to the area for no longer than 10 minutes
at a time, alternating 10 minutes on and 10 minutes off for an hour.
Before using ice, wrap the area with a wet elastic bandage.* The
bandage will help control swelling and the wet will speed the cold to the
tissue. If it is a foot that is injured, it should be elevated if possible to
assist in venous drainage and aid in healing.

Ice may be used several times—no longer than 10 minutes at a
time—for 48 to 72 hours following the injury. The muscle should be
rested until it is pain-free and a full range of use is regained. Then start

*Ice therapy also is effective if the pack is applied to dry skin. A light towel should be wrapped
around the bag to prevent possible tissue injury. Persons with circulatory problems should not use
any cold compress except as directed by a physician.

slowly but progressively to strengthen the injured muscle, but do not try to stretch it out for some time. Stretching should be done only after the muscle has been strengthened.

The efficacy of cryotherapy is well proven. The Air Force Academy makes extensive use of ice. *Fundamentals of Athletic Training,* a joint publication of the National Athletic Trainers Association, The Athletic Institute, and the A.M.A. Medical Aspects of Sports Committee, terms the treatment "of choice in managing the early stages of sprains, strains and contusions."

The sooner ice packs are used, the greater their control of pain and swelling, Drs. W. Bruce Conolly, N. Paltos, and R. M. Tooth of Sydney Hospital, Australia, have found. In their research they used Cryogel, a gel ice pack. Such packs as Cryogel, Cold/Hot Pack, and others are stored in the refrigerator freezer compartment, where they remain flexible and easily handled.

KNEE PROBLEMS

Many joggers believe they are the only ones who are bothered with chondromalacia, a wearing away of the back of the kneecap. But they are not alone; the problem also is found among competitive swimmers, bicycle riders, and gymnasts. It is a painful condition. Often there is a grating sensation behind the kneecap during walking, running, and climbing of stairs. There are a number of causes of chondromalacia, among them weak quadriceps (front of the thigh) muscles, kneecap/leg bone misalignment, improper running techniques, toeing out feet, poorly fitted shoes, and shoes that have been allowed to run down at the heels.

Some women only discover that they are bothered with foot imbalances and misalignments after they develop knee pains. Until they stressed their legs, they were unaware that these conditions existed. They also discover that one foot problem may lead to others, including heel bone bruises, irritation of the surface of the bottom of the foot, heel spurs, inflammation of the Achilles tendon, and nerve entrapment at the heel.

For many of these conditions, the best treatment is a cutting back of the number of miles run per week. But many addicted joggers refuse this remedy; they turn instead to store-bought orthotics (shoe inserts) or they buy another make of running shoe. Often, they discover the right combination of orthotic and shoe quickly and the pain subsides. Others find they must consult a sports-oriented podiatrist or orthopedist for help.

Of course, should surgery be recommended for any reason, another opinion should be sought. New advances in the use of orthotics have almost eliminated surgery from consideration for many foot problems.

FOOT CARE

The active woman's foot is susceptible to a wide variety of common conditions, such as athlete's foot, excessive sweating, corns, and calluses.

"Athlete's foot" is among the most common skin complaints seen by doctors. Originally it was considered to be caused entirely by a fungus. Today it is recognized that some infections between the toes are caused by bacteria.

The most common foot care problems include the following:

Tinea Pedis is found among basketball, tennis, and track players. The skin disease is caused by fungi and usually is spread through shower facilities and may be avoided by the wearing of sandals to reduce skin contact. The absorption of moisture by gym socks adds to the favorable conditions for fungal growth. An extra pair of socks should be kept in the gym bag or locker for immediate change when needed. Feet should be kept as dry as possible.

Candida Albicans, another bothersome foot problem which can involve the hands, also is common in running sports and swimming. Here too it is important to keep the feet dry after workouts. Dr. Sorrel S. Resnick, a Miami dermatologist, advises not to use foot powder containing starch, as starch actually is a nutrient for various fungi. He works with ZeaSorb, a nonstarch powder containing microporous cellulose which eliminates organism overgrowth.

Corns are caused by ill-fitting shoes and also are common to running sports. They are best treated by a podiatrist, who will use chemicals or minor surgery to remove the corns.

Plantar Callus is a buildup of the horny layers of the skin and it can easily be pared by a podiatrist. The use of special arch supports or foot pads to redistribute the weight is often recommended.

Tennis Toe is caused by the sudden stops that occur during a fast game. The toe bends and then hemorrhages under the nail. Tennis shoes built with a high toe cap help prevent this problem.

A number of these conditions are being successfully treated by the use of epidermabrasion (skin abrasion) by Dr. E. L. Cherniak, a Los Angeles podiatrist. He instructs his patients in the use of the nonmedicated Buf-Puf polyester cleansing pad which, when used daily, helps cure calloused heels, fissured areas, tinea pedis, and foot ulcers.

For many, foot care begins at home, not in the podiatrist's office. When publicist Lee Horn was researching various ways women athletes cared for their feet, she was told that marathoner Kathy Switzer uses Band-Aids to protect her toes from rubbing and blistering while she is running. Others said they used a moistened pumice stone on the tips of their toes to cope with calluses that may be forming there, and mentioned that pumice also is often effective when used on the ball of the foot.

If an area is particularly sensitive, a small moleskin suspension bridge can easily be made. Cut a hole in a small piece of moleskin and place it on the foot, with the hole surrounding the spot that hurts. Then lay a second moleskin over the first.

PERSONAL QUESTIONS WOMEN HAVE ABOUT EXERCISE

The Air Force Academy Women's Integration Research Project reported findings that exercise may help women suffering from dysmenorrhea, or painful menstruation. Other research has shown that overtraining may interrupt the normal rhythmic menstrual pattern. When exercise stress is reduced, there is a return to the previous rhythm.

How will regular exercise affect fertility? Would women have a greater chance of conceiving if they trained regularly?

Rena S. Bramnick has extensive experience in monitoring drug studies in women who do not ovulate, and in working with LH-RH, a pituitary-releasing hormone. She also was administrative director of the New York Fertility Research Foundation. Miss Bramnick says that the tremendous difficulties involved in measuring fertility as well as the complexities of doing controlled studies in this area make it unlikely these questions ever will be answered definitively. Should there be a noticeable up- or downturn in pregnancies in the next 20 to 25 years, some researchers may look to women's new interest in exercise for answers. But those answers of necessity must be generalized.

There is little question that pregnancy is no handicap to the active woman. Pregnant women run marathons, play tennis, swim regularly. Still the odds are that few obstetricians will permit a deconditioned pregnant woman suddenly to undertake vigorous exercise. If she has been active, there should be little reason for her not continuing as long as there is no danger of injuring her back or falling.

In general, women who are physically fit experience faster postpartum recoveries. Because exercise is an anti-depressant, they also should be able to cope better with the psychological problems posed by menopause.

Nutrition, Weight Control, and Allied Activities

Ponce de León searched for the fountain of youth. It's a quest many athletes still pursue, but they do not look for a fountain. Their search is for a powder, a pill, a potion that will give them extra energy and speed, that will help them win more than just a T-shirt or a mention in a program.

Before the advent of soaring meat prices and the question of cholesterol, college training tables were heaped high with steaks. The emphasis on meat was based on the premise that the more protein you ate, the stronger you would be and the more endurance you would have. That premise has been proved incorrect. Protein *is* important to health, but not critical to stamina or speed.

Fats and carbohydrates are used primarily for energy. During digestion, carbohydrates are changed to simple sugars or glucose. Liver cells take this glucose from the blood and convert it to glycogen. Glucose also is taken by the skeletal muscles and stored as glycogen until needed. It is this glucose converted into glycogen that energizes the body and muscles. Protein is used as an energy source only if glucose is not available. Excess carbohydrates that cannot be stored as glycogen in the liver and muscles are converted into fat.

GLYCOGEN OVERLOAD

Physiologists studying the causes of muscle fatigue found that lactic acid buildup; changes in the balance of sodium, potassium, and other electrolytes; heat overload; and poor cardiac reserve contributed to lack of muscular endurance.

173

The answer to the question of how to keep muscles energized eluded researchers until Dr. Per-Olaf Astrand, the noted physiologist, developed the carbohydrate or glycogen overload diet.

This diet called for endurance athletes to work to exhaustion about a week before a major event. This would burn off the glycogen normally stored in their muscles. They would then follow it with a low-carbohydrate diet for a period of three days and then switch to a high-carbohydrate regime. The deliberate depletion of glycogen followed by a high amount of carbohydrates "tricks" the body into overstuffing muscles with glycogen.

For marathoners who "hit the wall"—found themselves unable to energize their muscles at the 21-mile mark—carbohydrate overloading held out an answer to that problem by giving them the energy they needed to go the full 26 mile distance.

Today, the popularity of overloading appears to be waning. Some athletes found that the diet upset their systems. Others believe it is not necessary.

Dr. William P. Morgan, a consultant to various Olympic and national teams and a professor in the Department of Physical Education at the University of Arizona, finds that a number of world-class runners consider the wall a myth. Still others such as Dr. Elsworth R. Buskirk, director of the Laboratory for Human Performance Research at Pennsylvania State University, hold that most sports competition does not require glycogen loading. A number of women runners have commented that they believe women are impervious to the wall and the need for super-compensatory diets. One explanation given is that women burn protein more readily than men, so it is possible for them quickly to tap stored fat for energy.

YOUR BASIC DIET

Discussing the nutritional needs of athletes, Drs. Ralph A. Nelson and Clifford F. Gastineau of the Mayo Clinic and Mayo Foundation assert that high-protein, high-calorie diets; carbohydrate loading; vitamin supplements; and starvation are nutritional practices of athletes that are harmful or potentially harmful.

High-protein, high-calorie diets can produce obesity and shorten life span; carbohydrate loading can produce electrocardiographic abnormalities; vitamin supplements can be toxic; and starvation can adversely affect protein metabolism, blood volume, and athletic performance.

Observations of humans and experiments with animals indicate that the eating of fewer calories and less protein is more healthful. Protein and calorie restriction can double and even triple life span.

Many nutritionists agree that daily food requirements should be selected from the Basic Four: (1) milk group; (2) meat group; (3) vegetable-fruit group; (4) bread–cereal group.

> *Milk Group:* Skim, instant nonfat dry milk powder, buttermilk, nonfat pot cheese, cottage cheese, low-calorie American cheese.
> *Meat Group:* Lean meat, poultry, fish.
> *Vegetable–Fruit Group:* A citrus fruit or other Vitamin C-rich fruit or vegetable daily; dark leafy green or deep yellow vegetable for Vitamin A at least every other day. Drain heavily sugared syrups from canned fruits before using.
> *Bread–Cereal Group:* Whole-grain bread; sugar-free cereals. Beans, corn, potatoes, and dried peas belong in this group.

For snacking, keep already prepared in the refrigerator any of the following: radishes, celery, carrot sticks, green pepper sticks, cucumber slices.

Desserts are good for the soul, but the more often you say no to unnecessarily sweetened pastries and cakes, the more readily will you be able to control any weight problem you may have.

WEIGHT LOSS OR GAIN: LONG-TERM PROJECTS

Extra pounds in the form of flab indicate that food calories have been taken in faster than they have been burned up by physical activity. Underweight, if there is no underlying medical problem, indicates that the daily intake of food has been too low.

If the putting on of weight is advisable, the answer is to eat more, something that is difficult for many persons. Any increase in food intake should be made gradually, and in-between meals snacking may be advisable. Any woman suffering with anorexia—the absence or repression of appetite—should obtain professional care. The condition and accompanying weight loss may be caused by anemia or glandular deficiencies.

For many women, the American dream revolves around the concept of weight loss. But weight loss should be approached as a gradual, long-term project. The quick losses offered by crash and fad diets can prove harmful. Some women who go from fad diet to fad diet have weight records that look like a Yo-Yo.

An approach to weight loss that holds the promise of lasting success calls for (1) a reduction in calories, (2) a balanced diet, and (3) exercise.

Exercise burns up calories. If the calories are not supplied in excess by food, they will come from fat. Interestingly, exercise does not necessarily stimulate appetite. Because the obese woman has large stores of fat, moderate exercise will not stimulate her appetite. The lean woman soon will learn to balance her food intake with her exercise caloric "outgo."

ENERGY EXPENDITURE

Two brisk 15-minute walks a day can help you shed 10 pounds a year or keep you from putting them on. Couple this with a daily reduction of 250 calories in your diet, and you can lose more than 50 pounds in a year.

The more strenuous your exercise, the greater the number of calories you will consume. The calorie expenditure of different types of exercise has been established and is shown below. There are a number of variables that enter into these calculations, among them body weight and how strenuously you exercise. The figures shown for calorie expenditures are probably underestimates. The effects of exercise often continue after you have stopped. Body processes that have been increased are only gradually lowered, and this too takes energy.

Activity	Calorie cost per hour
Lying down or sleeping	80
Sitting	100
Driving an automobile	120
Standing	140
Doing Housework	180
Bicycling (5½ mph)	210
Walking (2½ mph)	210
Gardening	220
Canoeing (2½ mph)	230
Golf	250
Bowling	270

Activity	Calorie cost per hour*
Lawn mowing (hand mower)	270
Fencing	300
Rowboating (2½ mph)	300
Swimming (¼ mph)	300
Walking (3¾ mph)	300
Badminton	350
Horseback riding (trotting)	350
Volleyball	350
Roller skating	350
Table tennis	360
Ice skating (10 mph)	400
Tennis	420
Skiing (10 mph)	600
Cycling (13 mph)	660
Running (10 mph)	900

*This table shows energy cost per hour for a 150-pound person. To determine calorie expenditure for your weight, use the following formula:

$$\frac{\text{Activity cost shown above} \times \text{Your weight}}{150} = \text{Your energy expenditure}$$

IRON DEFICIENCY

Iron deficiency appears to be common among women. The mineral is a vital component of the red blood cells which carry oxygen from the lungs to the body. Its lack is usually readily corrected.

Normally women should be able to maintain their iron levels by including iron-rich foods in their diet—meat, especially liver; egg yolk; enriched and whole-grain bread and cereal; dried fruit; dried peas and beans; and leafy dark green vegetables.

If after tests your physician assures you that you do not need iron or other supplements, there is little need to take them "just to be safe."

SMOKING

Coaches have long been telling their charges that smoking cuts down the wind. Recent studies show that smoking has other effects. Blood plasma levels of Vitamin C in heavy smokers are up to 30 percent lower than in nonsmokers. British researchers studying groups of men and women found that smoking increases blood fat levels in both sexes. The increase was greater among women heavy smokers than among men, the blood cholesterol mean value reaching 239 for women and 184 for men.

ALCOHOL

It is doubtful anyone has successfully trained on alcohol for any period of time. Chronic heavy consumption of alcohol—wine contains alcohol, by the way—may interfere with the body's utilization of Vitamins B_1, B_6, and folic acid. An adequate supply of B_1 is needed for the maintenance of normal appetite and action of the digestive tract. A B_6 deficiency may lead to dermatitis. Folic acid functions in the maturation of red and white blood cells. Pernicious anemia and other anemias are treated by administering folic acid.

The problem of alcohol among women has surfaced alarmingly during the past few years. Edith Lynn Hornik, author of the informative *The Drinking Woman*, asserts that more women than men appear to take up drinking in desperation and out of loneliness. They also may be faced with unhappy family relationships or an unsuccessful marriage or both, leading to a loss of self-esteem.

A number of live-in treatment centers are using such sports as tennis and swimming, even calisthenics, to bolster self-esteem. As the alcoholic becomes increasingly adept at a sport, her belief in herself and her abilities is rebuilt. She gains confidence. This in addition to other rehabilitative efforts helps her to rebuild her life.

Mind Set

Women's minds often play games with them. First the mind urges them to start training. Then it presents a host of reasons why they should skip a session or not do that extra lap or mile.

Your ability to say no to your mind while you are accustoming it and yourself to a regular program of workouts can make the difference between successfully achieving your goals and having fun, or quitting.

Success in sports does not necessarily mean being able to run or swim marathons. Dr. Thomas Bassler, of the American Medical Joggers Association and an outspoken exponent of the belief that only the marathoner's lifestyle provides apparent immunity from coronary heart disease, admits that only a relatively small group through self-selection are able to impose that lifestyle's limitations on themselves.

Thousands of women set more limited goals for themselves. They are content with improving their physical abilities and cardiovascular reserve, and having fun. Achieving just these objectives requires enough dedication to help them surmount the initial mental and physical blocks to the point where working out becomes a positive addiction.

That takes weeks and often months, but once that point is reached, it often is the mind that inspires the lagging body. It is then that the body is castigated when a workout is missed. The mind needs and wants the workouts it has become accustomed or addicted to. In

179

his book *The Positive Addiction*, Dr. William Glasser touches on a result of the mentally relaxed state that is often achieved during training sessions. During these states the brain has an opportunity to grow and expand its horizons without restrictions—and without drugs.

SELF-MOTIVATION

Many women find all the motivation they need within themselves to begin running, swimming, or playing tennis. Others require stimulation and, on occasion, prodding. For these, there are a number of tested methods for keeping on schedule:

1. Train with a friend. If you set aside specific times to meet during the week, you become mutually self-supporting. This system works best if the other person needs little urging to exercise.

2. Join a running, canoeing, tennis, or other sports group. As you become involved, you make friends and exercise becomes a more enjoyable experience.

3. Set up a simple log in a notebook. Every page can cover a week's activities. Sections should be set up covering the amount of time spent during every workout, the distance covered and time spent, problems encountered. Several lines should be set aside for reasons why a session was missed. Any reason given must be valid to be accepted.

4. Set up a series of realistic objectives. Reaching them can become a goal in itself.*

5. Join a health club or gym. Many persons find they maintain a schedule only after making a monetary investment in what they are doing.

---

*The President's Council on Physical Fitness and Sports conducts an extensive program to encourage older youth and adults to remain physically active. The program emphasizes regular exercise rather than outstanding performance to maximize fitness benefits and enjoyment of sports. A log is supplied free to let you keep a record of your activity, and a Presidential Sports Award Certificate, emblem, and pin are presented to those completing the qualifications. Sports include archery, backpacking, badminton, basketball, biathlon, bicycling, bowling, canoe-kayak, climbing, equitation, fencing, figure skating, fitness walking, golf, gymnastics, handball, ice skating, jogging, judo, karate, orienteering, pentathlon, racquetball, rifle, roller skating, rowing, rugby, running, sailing, scuba-skin, skeet-trap, skiing (Alpine), skiing (Nordic), soccer, softball, squash, table tennis, team handball, tennis, volleyball, water skiing, weight training. For information write to the Presidential Sports Award, Greene, Rhode Island 02827.

STRESS AND DEPRESSION

Change is stressful—change in marital status, loss of job, changing to a different kind of work, foreclosure on a mortgage, or taking out a loan. Even successes cause stress.

Depression is a stress, something everyone suffers at times. It is a by-product of living and coping. That we get depressed is not as important as how we handle it, says psychiatrist Frederic F. Flach.

Many women I have trained with instinctively have turned to exercise to help them overcome depression caused by divorce or the death of a husband or child. For many years physicians have counseled patients to take walks to lift themselves out of depressions.

Now there appears to be a biological explanation for this phenomenon. In *The Secret Strength of Depression*, Dr. Flach cites a number of physiological changes that occur with states of depression.

In their work at the Payne Whitney Clinic, Dr. Flach and other researchers found that depressed patients who recovered after shock treatments showed a marked decrease in the urinary excretion of calcium and a significant increase in the amount of calcium retained by the body. This finding led to other questions, among them the question of whether regular physical activity, which is believed to be associated with an increase in calcium retention, works to counteract depression. Is regular physical activity of curative value in those already caught in chronic depression? Research now is going on in the areas of mineral metabolism, endocrine metabolism, the central-nervous-system transmitters, and genetic determinants relating to the manic-depressive condition.

At the University of Washington, Dr. Thomas H. Holmes and associates investigated the impact of life events and their role in such illnesses as colds, tuberculosis, and skin disease. Working from patients' responses, they listed and scored the events that patients most often cited as occurring before they became ill. Only some of the events were obviously negative, among them jail terms, sexual difficulties, death of spouses, being fired. Most were ordinary everyday events of life, such as visits by in-laws, going on vacation, being promoted.

Their studies showed that anyone scoring less that 150 points in the Schedule of Recent Experience (SRE) has only a one in three chance of serious health change in the following two years. If the score is between 150 and 300 points, chances of illness rise to about 50-50. Anyone scoring over 390 points is at extremely high risk.

SCHEDULE OF RECENT EXPERIENCE (SRE) *(Short Form)*

1. Under "Number of Occurrences" indicate how many times in the past year each of the events has occurred.

2. Multiply the number under "Scale Value" by the number of occurrences of each event and place the answer under "Your Score."

3. Add the figures under "Your Score" to find your total for the past year.

Life Event	Number of Occurrences	Scale Value	Your Score
Death of spouse	――	100	――
Divorce	――	73	――
Marital separation from mate	――	65	――
Detention in jail or other institution	――	63	――
Death of a close family member	――	63	――
Major personal injury or illness	――	53	――
Marriage	――	50	――
Being fired at work	――	47	――
Marital reconciliation with mate	――	45	――
Retirement from work	――	45	――
Major change in the health or behavior of a family member	――	44	――
Pregnancy	――	40	――
Sexual difficulties	――	39	――
Gaining a new family member (e.g., through birth, adoption, oldster moving in, etc.)	――	39	――
Major business readjustment (e.g., merger, reorganization, bankruptcy, etc.)	――	39	――
Major change in financial state (e.g., a lot worse off or a lot better off than usual)	――	38	――
Death of a close friend	――	37	――
Changing to a different line of work	――	36	――
Major change in the number of arguments with spouse (e.g., either a lot more or a lot less than usual regarding child-rearing, personal habits, etc.)	――	35	――
Taking on a mortgage greater than $10,000 (e.g., purchasing a home, business, etc.)	――	31	――
Foreclosure on a mortgage or loan	――	30	――
Major change in responsibilities at work (e.g., promotion, demotion, lateral transfer)	――	29	――

Life Event	Number of Occurrences	Scale Value	Your Score
Son or daughter leaving home (e.g., marriage, attending college, etc.)	————	29	————
In-law troubles	————	29	————
Outstanding personal achievement	————	28	————
Wife beginning or ceasing work outside the home	————	26	————
Beginning or ceasing formal schooling	————	26	————
Major change in living conditions (e.g., building a new home, remodeling, deterioration of home or neighborhood)	————	25	————
Revision of personal habits (dress, manners, associations, etc.)	————	24	————
Troubles with the boss	————	23	————
Major change in working hours or conditions	————	20	————
Change in residence	————	20	————
Changing to a new school	————	20	————
Major change in usual type and/or amount of recreation	————	19	————
Major change in church activities (e.g., a lot more or a lot less than usual)	————	19	————
Major change in social activities (e.g., clubs, dancing, movies, visiting, etc.)	————	18	————
Taking on a mortgage or loan less than $10,000 (e.g., purchasing a car, TV, freezer, etc.)	————	17	————
Major change in sleeping habits (a lot more or a lot less sleep, or change in part of day when asleep)	————	16	————
Major change in number of family get-togethers (e.g., a lot more or a lot less than usual)	————	15	————
Major change in eating habits (a lot more or a lot less food intake, or very different meal hours or surroundings)	————	15	————
Vacation	————	13	————
Christmas	————	12	————
Minor violations of the law (e.g., traffic tickets, jaywalking, disturbing the peace, etc.)	————	11	————

This is your total life change score for the past year ————

(For demonstration purposes only; not considered suitable for research.)

Dr. Thaddeus Kostrubala in *The Joy of Running* tells how a three times a week running-group psychotherapy had positive results in two studies. Individuals suffering with depression, schizophrenia, anorexia nervosa, and lifestyle changes had improved functioning. Dr. Kostrubala suggests that running immediately before psychotherapy "stimulates ... openings into the unconscious and is a valuable tool in the therapeutic process."

Other reports have told of running programs that often help patients recover from severe depressions following heart attacks.

Little, however, has been done on a controlled basis to study the effects of exercise—and specifically running—on depression. At the University of Wisconsin Dr. John H. Greist and five associates undertook such a study. Thirteen men and fifteen women patients were assigned randomly either to running or to one of two kinds of psychotherapy. Ten received running treatment, six got time-limited psychotherapy, and twelve received time-unlimited psychotherapy. Treatment continued for ten weeks. Patients were encouraged to run at least three times weekly either with the leader or alone. They were encouraged to become independent runners, capable of continuing self-treatment after the ten-week study ended.

At the end of ten weeks, six of the eight patients (two had dropped out) who ran for ten weeks had recovered from their depression. This compared with the best results generally obtained at the university clinic. Improvement in the runners often began during the first week and was usually substantial within three weeks.

Of course, more research is required to verify and amplify this study's findings. There is no evidence that running would be helpful in the management of major depressions that now are being managed by anti-depressant medications, shock, and other therapies.

Dr. Greist and his group of investigators evolved a number of hypotheses that may explain the beneficial effects running appears to have on depression. As a group, they highlight the psychological benefits enjoyed by runners, and often by those who participate regularly in other activities.

1. Mastery. Individuals who become independent runners develop a sense of success and mastery.
2. Patience. They relearn the necessity of patience and regular effort.
3. Capacity for change. They become aware they can change for the better, improving their health, appearance, and body image.

4. Generalization. Proving themselves competent in running helps them feel capable of becoming competent in other areas.
5. Distraction. Their minds are turned away from minor physical symptoms to the real sensations of sports.
6. Positive habit or "addiction." Activity becomes a positive substitute for negative habits.
7. Symptom relief. Running proves a reliable means of losing symptoms of anger and anxiety.
8. Consciousness alteration. Often associated with distance running, experienced runners describe this state as a positive, creative, less conscious, and more insightful interlude.
9. Biochemical changes. A number of investigators, including Dr. Flach as mentioned previously, are working in this area. Dr. Greist and his associates point out that "it seems certain that biochemical correlates of clinical depression will eventually be found."

YOU CAN BE IN CONTROL

Happily, most women are not forced to turn to sports for therapy. Still, most of us are buffeted from time to time and feel we are at the mercy of forces outside our control at work, in the home, or in our personal lives.

There are a number of ways we can marshal our thoughts to help us control our reactions to our environment. Dr. Florence Denmark, president of the American Psychological Association, reminds us that one of the ways we can stay in control of work situations is to improve our skills by attending training sessions, even by going back to school. We can also make up our minds that we are masters of our reactions to situations we are involved in; we can even decide at times to thrust problems out of our mind, to deny that the stress and tension exist, so long as we do not escape reality.

Often this is not a simple task, but it can be done as William Ernest Henley declared in the final lines of *Invictus*:

> It matters not how strait the gate,
>   How charged with punishments the scroll,
> I am the master of my fate;
>   I am the captain of my soul.

Appendix A: Personal Safety

There is no need to become paranoid, but the question of personal safety affects all sports and activities: personal flotation gear and the HELP position in boating safety; correctly fitted shoes for skiing, running, and hiking; protection against wind and chill in outdoor sports. Bicycles now must be sold with reflectors attached. For older vehicles there are easily installed inexpensive clip-on reflectors, and even tires with reflective tapes built into them. Some running shoes and other outdoor gear are made with reflective tape so the wearer can easily be seen in the glare of automobile headlights.

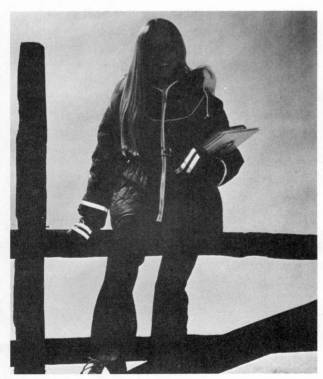

Reflective tape is being increasingly used on clothing, shoes, and packs to afford an extra margin of safety to hikers, runners, and others in the dark. (*3M photo*)

SEXUAL AGGRESSION*

Unfortunately, the problem of sexual aggression is real. There are reports of women being attacked while jogging or camping.

Total safety cannot be guaranteed for anyone; still there are basic safety guidelines every woman should be familiar with to put herself at low risk. One principle that is taught to Air Force Academy women cadets is to avoid hitchhiking. Only too often the end of the ride is grim—assault, robbery, rape, murder.

If you are jogging alone or cannot take a cab home at night, go out of your way to walk on well-lighted streets. If you must use a deserted street, walk in the center of the road. You will be able to see a car's headlights long before it nears you, so don't worry about being hit. Should a car pull up and start following you, immediately turn and run in the opposite direction. The driver must get out or make a U-turn if he is set on grabbing you. By then, you may be able to slip into a neighbor's home, a lobby, or a late-open store, or just outrun him.

At home, if there is a stranger at your lobby door waiting for you to unlock it, walk back out. If he is still there after a time, call the police. If someone you do not know is at the elevator waiting to go in with you, let him go up alone.

Before you enter the elevator, if possible, reach in and press your floor button. If the elevator light flashes "down" even after you've pressed your button, let the elevator go down to the basement and stop it on its return up. Then look to see if there is anyone in the elevator before you step in.

If when you reach your floor you see someone just standing there, get back into the elevator and go back down. Go to a neighbor's home, if possible, or call the building superintendent and have him go up with you.

Avoid confrontation; do not fight to save a handbag or purse, police officers advise. But what if you believe rape is the objective of aggression? Should you fight or submit?

There is no firm answer. "That is a question women will have to decide instinctively," Ida McKinney, a former Denver deputy sheriff and a court marshal, told me. "In our experience with forcible rape, we find most attackers use their hands to grab and subdue a woman. If

*Excerpts reprinted by permission of *Woman's Day Magazine.* Copyright ©1976 by CBS Publications, Inc.

you do get caught and decide to fight back, you must be ready and able to really hurt your attacker enough to put him out of action. If you cannot, you may find one of your best defenses is to 'faint,' to go completely limp."

According to Officer Liddon Griffith of the New York City Housing Police Department, every jailed rapist he has spoken with admitted he was disgusted at the thought of attacking a vomiting woman. Officer Griffith recommends thrusting your fingers down your throat to throw up.

The question of whether a woman should carry a weapon invariably comes up during community discussions about personal safety and crime. "That will depend largely on local law and a woman's own inclination," said Chief Richard Young of the Alameda, California, Police Department. He believes that a woman's own ability to scream for help may be her best defense. (Ever pragmatic, many officers suggest screaming "Fire" instead of "Help" or "Rape.") But if you are elderly and can't run, fight, or scream, what then? You may want to carry an inexpensive battery- or gas-powered hand alarm or even an old-fashioned hat pin. If you do, don't bury it deep in your bag when you are out alone at night. Keep the alarm or pin close at hand.

Easily carried weapons are aerosol dog repellents or sprays marked "Keep out of eyes." Recently an internationally known athlete used dog repellent on a man who grabbed at her while she was on a training run. She was able to keep going without breaking her stride.

Officer Griffith and others believe that if women are given the self-confidence and the training, they can physically fight off attackers.

Any system, to be effective, must be practiced until it becomes instinctive. There should be no need to think of what to do next. And you should be willing to use it to disable, to give you enough time to break and get away.

Appendix B:
Mail Order Sources

In many sections of the country, women may find it difficult to find an adequate variety of sports and outdoor equipment from which to make a selection. There are a number of mail order houses — in addition to Sears, Montgomery Ward and J. C. Penney — to turn to for help. They include:

Eddie Bauer, Inc.
15010 N.E. 36th Street
Redmond, WA 98052

L.L. Bean, Inc.
Freeport, ME 04033

Early Winters, Ltd.
110 Prefontaine Pl. S.
Seattle, WA 98104

Eastern Mountain Sports
2310 Vose Farm Rd.
Peterborough, NH 03458

Frostline Kits
Frostline Circle
Denver, CO 80241

Don Gleason's Campers Supply, Inc.
20 Pearl Street
Northampton, MA 01060

Holubar Mountaineering, Ltd.
P.O. Box 7
Boulder, CO 80306

Morsan
P.O. Box 218
Paramus, NJ 07652

Sportswares
1155 Triton Drive
Foster City, CA 94404

Starting Line Sports
P.O. Box 8
Mt. View, CA 94042

Tough Traveler
1328 State Street
Schenectady, NY 12304

Waters, Inc.
111 E. Sheridan Street
Ely, MI 55731

Wilderness Concepts
4852 Laurel Canyon Blvd.
Hollywood, CA 91607

Notes & Readings

Preface
Anderson, L. H., Interview, October 1978.
Bernstein, B., "The Forgotten Women of World War II," *Daily News*, September 7, 1976.
Langford, D. L., "The Wasps of World War II: America's Forgotten Heroines," United Press International, September 12, 1976.
Strother, D. D., "The Wasp Training Program," *Journal American Aviation Historical Society*, Winter 1974.

Chapters 1–2
USAF Academy, Department of Physical Education: Women's Integration Research Project. Phase I, November 23, 1975; Phase II, April 27, 1977; Phase III, April 10, 1978.
———, Exercise demonstrations, July 1977, April 1978.

Chapter 3
Lasco, J. R., Personal communication, May 6, 1971.

Chapter 4
Exercise prescriptions, Cardio-Metrics Institute, September, 1978. Training effect pulse rates, Cardio-Metrics Institute, September 1978.

Chapter 5
"Comes the Revolution ... Women are Transforming American Athletics," *Time*, June 26, 1978.
Kevles B., Official Program, New York City Marathon, 1977.
USAF Academy, Department of Athletics, Athletic Training Summaries, May 1978.
"The Weaker Sex? Hah!" *Time*, June 26, 1978.
Young, K., "Best of Times," *Runner's World*, December 1976.

Chapter 6
Adult Physical Fitness, President's Council on Physical Fitness, 1965.
Bengtsson, H., and G. Atkinson, *Orienteering for Sport and Pleasure*, The Stephen Greene Press, 1977.
Borkowski, R., "Wall to Wall Circuit Training," Fitness for Living, September/October 1970.
Carlton, C. K., The Many Curves of Eve," paper, The American Osteopathic Association national convention, 1976.

Galub, J., "Hiking," *Self* magazine, forthcoming.
Kjellström, B., *Be Expert With Map and Compass*, Charles Scribner's Sons, 1976.
Pamilla, J., Interview, 1977.
Youth Physical Fitness, President's Council on Physical Fitness and Sports, September 1973.
Zonana, V. F., "Publishers, lured by 'great demographics,' rush to put our magazines for joggers and runners," *The Wall Street Journal*, April 28, 1978.

Chapter 7
Blocker, W. P., Jr., "Physical Activities," *Postgraduate Medicine*, August 1976.
Castello, H., and J. Castello, *Fencing*, The Ronald Press Company, 1962.
Galub, J., "Our Newest Sport: Ski Camping," *Mechanix Illustrated*, December 1976.
————, "The Pedal Pushers," *American Girl*, May 1971.
————, "Saddle Up! Ride Your Bike for Fun and Health," *House Beautiful*, April 1971.
Hlavaty, J., Interview, August 1978.
Law, D., *The Beginner's Guide to Swimming and Water Sports*, Drake Publishers, Inc., 1975.
Lederer, W. J., and J. P. Wilson, *Complete Cross-Country Skiing and Ski Touring*, W. W. Norton & Co., 1970.
Lund, M., et al., *Ski Magazine's Complete Book of Ski Technique*, Harper & Row, 1975.
McCulloch, E., *Ski Easy ... The New Technique*, McGraw-Hill Ryerson Ltd., 1973.
Russell, C. W., *Basic Canoeing*, The American National Red Cross, 1963.
Schroeder, B., Interview, July 1977.
Stark, M., "What Do You Mean, You Don't Have a Paddling Partner," *Wilderness Camping's Canoe & Kayak '78*, 1978.

Chapter 9
Astrand, P. O., *Health and Fitness*, Scandia Insurance Co., Ltd., Swedish Information Service, 1973.
Astrand, P. O., and K. Rodahl, *Textbook of Work Physiology*, McGraw-Hill, 1970
Benson, H., *The Relaxation Response*, William Morrow & Co., 1975.
Blakeslee, A., and J. Stamler, *Your Heart Has Nine Lives*, Prentice-Hall, Inc., 1963.
Chapman, A. H., *Textbook of Clinical Psychiatry*, J. P. Lippincott Co., 1967.
"Detection, Evaluation and Treatment of High Blood Pressure," U.S. Department of Health, Education and Welfare, National Heart, Lung, and Blood Institute, 1977, *Medical Times*, May 1978.
deVries, H. A., *Laboratory Experiments in Physiology of Exercise*, W. C. Brown, 1971.
Finnerty, F., Jr., "The Problem of Non-compliance," *Medical Times*, May 1978.
Friedman, M., and R. H. Rosenman, *Type A Behavior and Your Heart*, Alfred A. Knopf, 1974.
Fries, E. D., "A Complete Guide to (Hypertension) Drug Treatment," *Medical Times*, May 1978.
Galub, J., "Keep Your Heart in Shape with CVT," *Retirement Living*, April 1975.

————, "Rx Pep for a Full Life," North Shore University Hospital, Cardio-Metrics Institute, 1976.

————, "Why Take a Stress Test?" *Runner's World*, October 1974.

Getchell, B., *Physical Fitness: A Way Of Life*, John Wiley & Sons, 1976.

Gitlin, E., "Controlling High Blood Pressure: The Nurse's Role," *American Journal of Nursing*, May 1978.

Gray, H., *Anatomy, Descriptive and Surgical*, Bounty Books, 1977.

Gualtiere, W. S., A. J. Delman and R. J. Becker, "The 'All-or-None' Law for Cardiovascular Enhancement," *The Daily Supplement*, undated.

Halberstam, M., and L. Lesher, *A Coronary Event*, Popular Library, 1978.

Heart Attack, American Heart Association, 1970.

Kannel, W. B. "Further Findings from Framingham," *Medical Times*, May 1978.

Katch, F. I., and W. D. McArdle, *Weight Control and Exercise*, Houghton Mifflin Company, 1977.

Kuntzleman, C. T., *The Physical Fitness Encyclopedia*, Rodale Books, Inc., July 1971.

Miller, B. F., L. Galton, and D. Brunner, *Freedom From Heart Attacks*, Simon & Schuster, 1972.

Simonelli, C., and R. E. Eaton, "Cardiovascular and Metabolic Effects of Exercise: The Strong Case for Conditioning," *Postgraduate Medicine*, February 1978.

Tobian, L., "What We Know About (Hypertension) Basic Mechanisms," *Medical Times*, May 1978.

Ward, G. W., P. Bandy, and J. W. Fink, "Treating and Counseling the Hypertensive Patient," *American Journal of Nursing*, May 1978.

"Widow, 75, Finds Backpacking Beats Rocking Chair in a Walk," *Grit*, June 11, 1978.

Wilson, D. L., *Total Mind Power*, Camaro Publishing Co., 1976.

"World's Quickness Fitness Test," *Medical Dimensions*, August/September 1973.

Chapter 10

Elliott, P. R., and H. A. Atterbom, "Comparison of Exercise Responses of Males and Females during Acute Exposure to Hypobaria," *Aviation, Space and Environmental Medicine*, February 1978.

————, Interviews, July 1977, April 1978.

Gieseking, H., "Six Simple Steps to Survival," *The Travel Advisor*, July 1977.

Hayward, J. S., M. L. Collis, and J. D. Eckerson, *Man in Cold Water*, The University of Victoria, 1975.

"Hypothermia and Cold Water Survival," Department of Transportation, U.S. Coast Guard, October 1976.

Knochel, J. F., Personal communication, The University of Texas Southwestern Medical School at Dallas, July 1977.

Price, D. L., "Overdrink for Survival," *Marine Corps Gazette*, June 1978.

Smith, D. S., "The Cold Water Connection," paper.

————, U. S. Coast Guard, Personal communication.

U.S. Army Natick Development Center, Various data, 1976, 1975.

U.S. Army Training Circular, No. 90-6-1, September 1976.

Chapter 11

Cherniak, E. L., "Epidermabrasion of the Foot," *Current Podiatry*, January 1976.

Conolly, W. B., N. Paltos, and R. M. Tooth, "Cold Therapy: An Improved Method," *The Medical Journal of Australia*, August 19, 1974.

Donahue, S., "Health: Sports/Women," *Vogue*, March 1978.

Downey, J. A., R. C. Darling, and J. M. Miller, "The Effects of Heat, Cold, and Exercise on the Peripheral Circulation," *Archives of Physical Medicine and Rehabilitation*, June 1968.

Eisenberg, I., and W. C. Allen, "Injuries in a Women's Varsity Athletic Program," *The Physician and Sportsmedicine*, March 1978.

Resnik, S. S., L. A. Lewis, and B. H. Cohen, *The Athlete's Foot*, University of Miami School of Medicine, 1977.

Seder, J. I., "Heel Injuries Incurred in Running and Jumping," *The Physician and Sportsmedicine*, October 1976.

Wilson, H., Personal communication, 1978.

Chapter 12

Buskirk, E. R., "Diet and Athletic Performance," *Postgraduate Medicine*, January 1977.

Denmark, F., Stress Seminar, City University of New York, Graduate Center, October 18, 1978.

Exercise and Weight Control, A.M.A. Committee on Exercise and Physical Fitness; President's Council on Physical Fitness; Lifetime Sports Foundation.

"Four Steps to Weight Control," Metropolitan Life Insurance Company, 1969.

HEW Study Finds Women Pay a Price for Smoking More, *Wall Street Journal*, undated.

Hornik, E. L., Personal communication, August 1978.

———, *The Drinking Woman*, Association Press, 1977.

Miller, M. A., and L. C. Leavell, *Anatomy and Physiology*, Macmillan Publishing Co., 1972.

Morgan, W. P., "The Mind of the Marathoner," *Psychology Today*, April 1978.

Nelson, R. A., and C. F. Gastineau, "Exceptional Nutritional Needs of the Athlete," 15th National Conference on the Medical Aspects of Sports, December 1973.

Nutrition for Athletes, American Association for Health, Physical Education, and Recreation, 1971.

Watt, B. K., et al, *Composition of Foods: Raw, Processed, Preapred, Consumer and Food Economics Institute*, U.S. Department of Agriculture, 1975.

Chapter 13

Flach, F. F., Personal communication, August 1978.

———, *The Secret Strength of Depression*, Bantam Psychology Books, 1974.

Galub, J., "Jog Anyone?" *Mothers' Manual*, June 1975.

Greist, J. H., et al, "Antidepressant Running," *Behavioral Medicine*, June 1978.

———, "Running as Treatment for Depression," University of Wisconsin-Madison, paper.

Holmes, T. H., Schedule of Recent Experience, 1976.

———, Stress seminar, Hotel Roosevelt, New York City, May 1978.

Holmes, T. H., and T. S. Holmes, "How Change Can Make Us Ill," *Stress*, Blue Cross Association, 1974.

Holmes, T. H. and M. Masuda, "Life Change and Illness Susceptibility," AAAS 1973, Publication No. 94.

Kostrubala, T., *The Joy of Running*, J. B. Lippincott, 1976.

Appendix

Galub, J., "Playing It Safe," *Woman's Day*, June 1973.

———. "You Can Protect Yourself," *Woman's Day*, September 1976.

Griffith, L., Interview, 1976.

McKinney I., Personal communication, interview, 1973, 1976.

Young, R., Personal communication, 1973.

Acknowledgments

There are many individuals, organizations, and corporations who were generous in providing me with essential research.

Military: I am indebted to Colonel Don L. Peterson, head of the Air Force Academy Department of Physical Education, for his guidance and Foreword, and to Major Philip R. Elliott for his comments and suggestions.

Captain Sherry Smith, First Lieutenant Darlene Riding, and Gail Lenneville went beyond the call of duty several times to demonstrate exercises for the photographs used here.

In New York City, Air Force Lieutenant Colonel Tom Maypole provided invaluable assistance in ferreting out needed materials and providing guidance.

Despite my focus on the Air Force Academy, members of other branches of the military were helpful, among them Major David Hague, Marine Corps, and Lieutenant Commander D. S. Smith, Coast Guard.

Government: A number of government agencies cooperated in making research available. Among them were the President's Council on Physical Fitness and Sports; Public Health Service; Food and Drug Administration; and the Agricultural Research Service.

Professional Groups: Nongovernmental organizations that were generous with research materials included The American Association for Health, Physical Education, and Recreation; National Academy of Sciences; and The University of Texas Health Science Center at Dallas.

Individuals: I am grateful to William S. Gualtiere, Ph.D., director of the Cardio-Metrics Institute in New York City, for his comments on cardiovascular fitness and Foreword, and to Phyllis Melhado for her willingness to be photographed while being exercise stress-tested.

There are many individuals who shared their knowledge and experience with me. Among them: Olympian Anne Henning, canoe/kayak experts Molly Stark and Bruce Schroeder, United States and

Czechoslovakia cross-country skiing champion Jana Hlavaty, fencer Priscilla DeMarinis and her instructor Miklos Bartha, and athletic trainer Holly Wilson.

Also: osteopathic physician Dr. Kenney Carlton; orthopedic surgeon Dr. Jeanne R. Pamilla; cardiologist Dr. Borisse B. Paulin; psychiatrists Dr. Frederic F. Flach, Dr. Thomas H. Holmes, and Dr. John H. Greist; Janaffa Brodie, R.N., and medical researcher Rena Bramnick.

Industry: Fripp Island, Service Corp., South Carolina; Killington, Vermont; Keystone, Colorado; 3M Company; Riker Laboratories; Stiefel Laboratories; Xerox Corporation, and others made photographs, charts, and other data available for use.

Prentice-Hall: The editorial and art departments were especially helpful. I should like to thank my editor, John Grayson Kirk, for his assistance and guidance, and editor Roy Winnick for his encouragement and patience.

I also wish to thank the many hundreds of exercise physiologists, cardiologists, trainers, and researchers upon whose shoulders I stood to write this book, as well as the Air Force Academy women cadets whose contributions to our country and this book can never be fully measured.

The Women's Integration Research Project Phase I report was written by Lieutenant Colonel James C. Thomas, D.P.E.; Captain Richard W. Coté III, M.A.; Captain Robert J. Zande, M.A.; Lieutenant Darlene E. Riding, M.S.; and then Captain Philip R. Elliott, Ph.D. The project originator was Colonel K. Strickland, then Head of the Physical Education Department at the Air Force Academy.

The project was begun on November 23, 1975, and submitted on December 17, 1976.

The same group wrote the Phase II report, which was submitted on April 20, 1977.

Phase III was prepared by Lieutenant Colonel James C. Thomas, D.P.E.; Major Harold M. Koerber, B.S.; Major Paul K. Maruyama, B.S.; Captain Robert E. Lushbaugh, B.S.; Lieutenant Darlene E. Riding, M.S.; Captain Charles P. Patton, M.S.; and Major Philip R. Elliott, Ph.D. The report was submitted on April 10, 1978.

Index

201

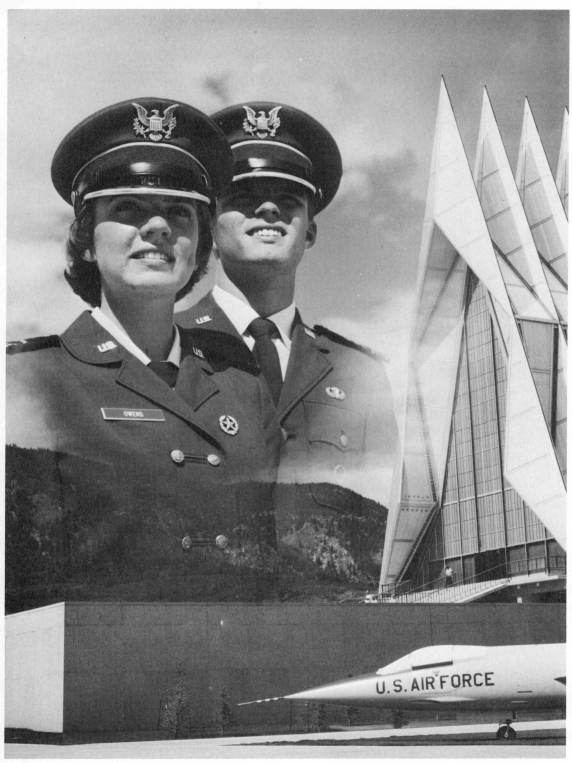

(Photograph courtesy of U.S. Air Force Academy)